Children's Spinal Disorders and Fractures

Michael Benson • John Fixsen • Malcolm Macnicol
Klaus Parsch
Editors

Children's Spinal Disorders
and Fractures

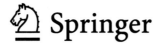 Springer

Editors

Michael Benson
Ridgway
Harberton Mead
OX3 ODB Oxford
United Kingdom
michael.benson@doctors.org.uk

John Fixsen
West Barn
Clamok Farm Barns
Wier Quay
PL20 7BU Bere Alston
United Kingdom
jafixsen@btinternet.com

Malcolm Macnicol
Red House
Gillsland Road 1
EH10 5DE Edinburgh
United Kingdom
mmacnicol@aol.com

Klaus Parsch
Weinbergweg 68
70569 Stuttgart Baden-
Württemberg
Germany
kparsch@t-online.de

ISBN 978-0-85729-557-6   e-ISBN 978-0-85729-558-3
DOI 10.1007/978-0-85729-558-3
Springer London Dordrecht Heidelberg New York

British Library Cataloguing in Publication Data
A catalogue record for this book is available from the British Library

Library of Congress Control Number: 2011929877

Cover design: eStudio Calamar S.L.

Printed on acid-free paper

Springer is part of Springer Science+Business Media (www.springer.com)

Foreword

Confirming the British genetic trait for writing and publishing (as well as acting), two English (Oxford and London) and a Scottish orthopaedic surgeon (Edinburgh) have produced a third edition of their comprehensive text, joined, as in the second edition by an editor from Germany, recognizing its part in the European community. The 62 physician contributors are drawn from pink-colored countries in our childhood geography books—the old British Empire from Australia to Zambia and two from the former colony, the USA.

The original purpose of the book was to give residents or registrars an easily accessible and concise description of diseases and conditions encountered in the practice of paediatric orthopaedic surgery and to prepare for their examinations. But the practicing orthopaedic surgeon will find an update of current practice that can be read for clarity and constraint—enough but not too much. A foreword might be a preview of things to come, but a "back word" of what was thought to be the final say on the subject is needed for a perspective in progress.

A "back word" look reveals the tremendous progress in medical diagnosis and treatment of which paediatric orthopaedics and fracture care is a component. Clubfoot treatment based on the dictums of Hiram Kite has had a revolutionary change by Ponseti. The chapter by Eastwood has the details on cast application and orthotics follow-up to obtain the 95% correction without the extensive surgery many of us thought was needed.

Paediatric fracture care has also changed from traction for fractures of the femoral shaft in the ages of 5–15 years to intramedullary fixation with elastic stable nails originated in Nancy and Metz, France—"Nancy nails." Klaus Parsch's chapter tells us that it is their preferred method of treatment in Stuttgart, Germany.

Robert Dickson's lucid writing on idiopathic scoliosis as primarily a rotation of the lordotic thoracic spine again bears study to deepen the understanding that it is a three-dimensional deformity. As in the past editions, a coat hanger helps to appreciate the distortion of curvatures in a one-dimensional radiograph. Those orthopaedists who need courage to resist pressure to encase children in casts or braces or orthoses will be heartened to know that none of these conservative measures have shown any effect in prevention or curve progression. What to do instead of "treatment"? Read on.

This is not a book to learn the details of surgical technique–other texts and only experience can do that. Even though a seasoned orthopaedic surgeon does not need this knowledge to pass an examination, he or she is expected to know something about the subject. Once identified as an orthopaedic surgeon, your opinion is often sought at social events usually standing with a drink in hand. And commonly it is advice sought by your married children about a grandchild's musculoskeletal problem. Can you answer sensibly? If, "I'll get back to you later" is your response, a quick perusal of the contents of this volume should help maintain your professional standing and as is now the fashion of school teachers, your "self-esteem." And you won't have to log on to the Internet.

Eugene E Bleck

Preface

This section brings together the congenital, acquired and traumatic conditions which may affect the child's cervical and thoraco-lumbar spine. The immature spine poses considerable diagnostic dilemmas and radiographs are often difficult to interpret. The aetiology of deformity, its assessment, monitoring and treatment are comprehensively described. Back pain in children receives special attention. Care has been taken to identify symptoms and signs which should raise our level of anxiety and those which are likely to resolve. Where surgery is necessary the principles and risks are defined.

Michael KD Benson, Oxford, UK   John A Fixsen, London, UK
Malcolm F Macnicol, Edinburgh, UK   Klaus Parsch, Stuttgart, Germany

June, 2011

Contents

Contributors

Clifford L. Craig Department of Orthopaedic Surgery, University of Michigan, Ann Arbor, MI, USA

Robert A. Dickson Academic Unit of Orthopaedic Surgery, Leeds General Infirmary, Leeds, UK

Robert N. Hensinger Department of Orthopaedic Surgery, University of Michigan, Ann Arbor, MI, USA

Chapter 1

Congenital Disorders of the Cervical Spine

Robert N. Hensinger

Radiological interpretation of the infant's spine may be difficult and a clear understanding of its appearance at different ages is essential if deformity and malalignment are to be recognized. Normal development of the cervical spine is discussed in the section on cervical trauma.

In 1912, Klippel and Feil [1] published the first description of various congenital disorders of the cervical spine. The "Klippel–Feil syndrome" in its present usage refers to all patients with congenital fusion of the cervical vertebrae, whether it involves two segments, congenital block vertebrae, or the entire cervical spine. As radiographic techniques improved, it became apparent that certain anomalies of the occipito-cervical junction, atlanto-occipital fusion, basilar impression, and abnormalities of the odontoid should be considered separately from the original syndrome. Although they occur commonly in conjunction with fusion of the lower cervical vertebrae, their significance depends upon their influence on the atlanto-axial joint. Their prognostic and therapeutic implications are distinctly different and they occur with sufficient frequency to warrant individual analysis.

Basilar Impression

Basilar impression (or basilar invagination) is a deformity of the bones of the base of the skull at the margin of the foramen magnum, The floor of the skull appears to be indented by the upper cervical spine. The tip of the odontoid is more cephalad, sometimes protruding into the opening of the foramen magnum, and it may encroach upon the brain-stem. This increases the risk of neurological damage from injury, circulatory embarrassment, or impairment of cerebrospinal fluid flow. There are two types:

1. Primary basilar impression. A congenital abnormality often associated with other vertebral defects such as atlanto-occipital fusion, hypoplasia of the atlas, bifid posterior arch of the atlas, odontoid abnormalities, and the Klippel–Feil syndrome.
2. Secondary basilar impression. A developmental condition attributed to softening of the osseous structures at the base of the skull, with deformity developing later in life. This occurs in conditions such as osteomalacia, rickets, Paget's disease, osteogenesis imperfecta, renal osteodystrophy, rheumatoid arthritis, neurofibromatosis, and ankylosing spondylitis.

Clinical Features

Patients with basilar impression frequently have a deformity of the skull or neck; however, these physical findings are also often found in patients without such impression (Klippel–Feil syndrome, occipitalization) and are not considered pathognomonic.

Basilar impression is often associated with conditions such as the Arnold–Chiari malformation and syringomyelia, which may cloud the clinical picture. Symptoms are generally caused by crowding of the neural structures (particularly the medulla oblongata) at the level of the foramen magnum. The dominant complaints of symptomatic patients are weakness and paresthesia of the limbs. In contrast, those who are symptomatic with pure Arnold–Chiari malformation are more likely to have cerebellar and vestibular disturbances (unsteadiness of gait, dizziness, and nystagmus). In both conditions, there may be impingement of the lower cranial nerves as they emerge from the medulla oblongata. The trigeminal (V), glossopharangeal (IX), vagus (X), and hypoglossal (X1I) nerves may be affected. Headache and pain in the nape of the neck in the distribution of the greater occipital nerve is a common finding. Posterior encroachment may cause blockage of the aqueduct of Silvius and the presenting symptoms may be caused by increased intracranial pressure [2].

R.N. Hensinger (✉)
Department of Orthopaedic Surgery, University of Michigan, Ann Arbor, MI, USA

There is an increased incidence of vertebral artery anomalies in basilar impression, atlanto-occipital fusion, and absence of the C1 facet. In addition, the vertebral arteries may be compressed as they pass through the crowded foramen magnum, causing symptoms suggestive of vertebral artery insufficiency, such as dizziness, seizures, mental deterioration, and syncope. These symptoms may occur alone or in combination with those of spinal cord compression. Erbengi and Oge [3] have noted that the preoperative evaluation of these patients needs special care as many have an unrecognized low vital capacity with chronic alveolar hypoventilation as a result of chronic slow progressive brainstem neurological injury. The gag and cough reflexes are often depressed.

Although this condition is congenital, many patients do not develop symptoms until the second or third decade. This may be due to a gradually increasing instability from ligamentous laxity. Patients with this malformation have been mistakenly diagnosed as having multiple sclerosis, posterior fossa tumors, amyotrophic lateral sclerosis or traumatic injury. It is therefore important to survey this area whenever such a diagnosis is considered and whenever this malformation is suspected.

Imaging Features

Basilar impression is difficult to assess radiographically and many measurement schemes have been proposed. The most commonly used are those described by Chamberlain [4], McGregor [5], and McRae [2]. McRae's line [2] defines the opening of the foramen magnum and is derived from his observation that "if the tip of the odontoid lies below the opening of the foramen magnum, the patient will probably be asymptomatic." It proves a helpful guide in the radiological assessment of patients with basilar impression (Fig. 1.1).

With the development of computed tomography (CT) reconstruction and, more recently, magnetic resonance imaging (MRI), it is now possible to view the relationship at the occipital-cervical junction in much greater detail [6, 7]. Clinically, the lateral reference lines [2, 5] are still important for screening. CT reconstruction and MRI are generally reserved for the patient whose routine examination or clinical findings suggest the presence of an occipito-cervical anomaly. Rouvreau et al. [8] found that occipital and atlas abnormalities were often associated with neurological risk. MRI with lateral flexion/extension views seems the best method of detecting spinal impingement on the spinal cord, especially in patients with odontoid dysplasia and basilar impression.

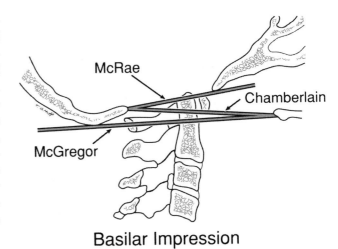

Basilar Impression

Fig. 1.1 Lateral craniometry. The drawing indicates the three lines used to determine basilar impressions. Chamberlain's line (1939) is drawn from the posterior lip of the foramen magnum (opisthion) to the dorsal margin of the hard palate. McGregor's line [5] is drawn from the upper surface of the posterior edge of the hard palate to the most caudal point of the occipital magnum. McGregor's line is the best method for screening, because the bony landmarks can be clearly defined at all ages on a routine lateral radiograph

Occipito-Cervical Fusion

Occipito-cervical fusion, which may be partial or complete, is a congenital union between the atlas and the base of the occiput. Synonyms include assimilation of the atlas, occipito-cervical synostosis, and occipitalization of the atlas. The condition ranges from total incorporation of the atlas into the occipital bone, to a bony or even fibrous band uniting one small area of the atlas to the occiput. Basilar impression is commonly associated with occipito-cervical synostosis. Other associated anomalies include the Klippel–Feil syndrome, occipital vertebrae, and condylar hypoplasia.

Clinical Features

Most patients have an appearance similar to the Klippel–Feil syndrome, with a short broad neck, low hairline, torticollis [6], high scapula, and restricted neck movements. Kyphosis and scoliosis are frequent. Other associated anomalies occasionally seen include dwarfism, funnel chest, pes cavus, syndactylies, jaw anomalies, cleft palate, congenital ear deformities, hypospadias, and genitourinary tract defects.

Neurological symptoms do not usually occur until middle life but they may present in childhood. They progress in a slow, unrelenting manner which may be initiated by trauma or an inflammatory process. Gholve et al. [6] recommend continued periodic clinical and radiographic evaluation because instability may occur with aging. McRae [2] suggested that the odontoid is the key to the development of a neurological lesion and that its position indicates the degree of actual or relative basilar impression. If the odontoid lies below the foramen magnum, the patient is usually asymptomatic. However, with decreased vertical height of the atlas, the odontoid may project well into the foramen magnum and produce brain-stem pressure. In children and adolescents with the Klippel–Feil syndrome, superior migration of the odontoid does not always correlate with symptoms. Those with four or more fused segments and, to a lesser degree, the female sex may have a higher risk of severe odontoid migration [9]. Fusion should be considered for those with instability and when signs of impingement on the spinal cord, nerve roots, or cranial nerves occur.

Anterior compression of the brain-stem from the posteriorly unstable odontoid is the most common problem. The neurological findings depend on the location and degree of pressure. Pyramidal tract symptoms and signs (spasticity, hyperreflexia, muscle weakness and wasting, and gait disturbances) are most common; cranial nerve involvement (diplopia, tinnitus, dysphagia, and auditory disturbances) is less common. Compression from the posterior lip of the foramen magnum or a constricting band of dura may disturb the posterior columns, resulting in loss of proprioception, vibration, and tactile discrimination. Nystagmus, a common occurrence, is probably due to posterior cerebellar compression. Vascular disturbances from vertebral artery involvement may occasionally result in syncope, seizure, vertigo, and unsteady gait among other signs and symptoms of brain-stem ischemia.

Imaging

Standard radiographs of this area can be difficult to interpret. CT reconstruction may be necessary to clarify the pathology. Most commonly, the anterior arch of the atlas is assimilated into the occiput, usually in association with a hypoplastic posterior arch. Congenital anomalies of the atlantal arch are usually incidental findings in asymptomatic patients. Congenital defects in the posterior arch are more common than those in the anterior arch [10]. There is varying loss of height of the atlas, allowing the odontoid to project upward into the foramen magnum and creating a primary basilar impression (Fig. 1.2). Gholve et al. [6] reviewed patients with occipitalization and identified four patterns of fusion:

- Zone 1—fused at the anterior arch
- Zone 2—fusion of the facets (lateral masses)
- Zone 3—fused at the posterior arch
- and a combination of these zones

There is a high association (up to 70%) with congenital fusion between C2 and C3, which can put added strain on the C1–C2 articulation (associated atlanto-axial instability has been reported to develop eventually in 50% of patients). CT reconstructions and MRI are important in establishing the diagnosis, assessing the zone of fusion, and measuring the encroachment [6].

Anomalies of the Ring of C1

In 1986, in the first large study, Dubousset [11] called attention to a previously barely recognized problem with the ring of C1, the hemi-atlas. The absence of one facet of C1 leads to a severe progressive torticollis in the young child. Initially, the deformity is flexible and can be passively corrected. As the child ages, the torticollis becomes more severe and eventually fixed. Radiographic diagnosis using tomograms or CT has helped to identify this deformity (Fig. 1.3), which may accompany the Klippel–Feil syndrome. Dubousset [11] found some of these children had associated anomalies of the vertebral vessels. He suggested arteriographic evaluation

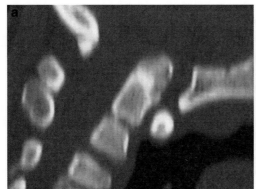
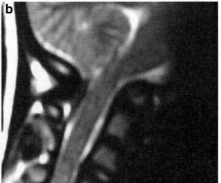

Fig. 1.2 A 10-year-old male with the Klippel–Feil syndrome. The lateral CT scan (**a**) and MRI (**b**) of the cervical spine and base of the skull demonstrate a C2–C3 fusion and odontoid protrusion into the opening of the foramen magnum. Patients with this pattern of fusion are at great risk. With aging the odontoid may become hypermobile, and the space available for the spinal cord may be compromised

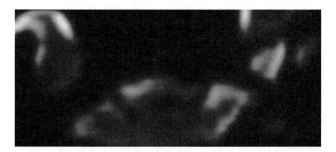

Fig. 1.3 Absent facet of C1: anteroposterior CT scan in a 5-year-old with a hemi-atlas that has led to a progressive torticollis. The deformity is initially flexible and passively correctible. Note that the left C1 facet is fused to the occiput

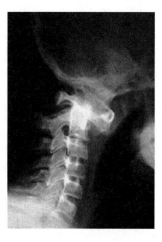

Fig. 1.4 The cervical spine of an 11-year-old with Down's syndrome and gross atlanto-axial instability. The gait was clumsy and physical examination revealed poor coordination of the extremities. There was no other evidence of motor or sensory impairment or of pathological reflexes. The patient has no symptoms referable to the cervical spine 2 years after surgical stabilization

before traction or surgical intervention, which could further compromise a precarious blood supply to the midbrain and spinal cord.

Laxity of the Transverse Atlantal Ligament

This is a diagnosis of exclusion suggested by the clinical occurrence of chronic atlanto-axial dislocation without a predisposing cause. There is no history of trauma, congenital anomaly, infection, or rheumatoid arthritis to account for the radiological finding. Most patients discovered (excluding those with Down's syndrome) have the typical symptoms of atlanto-axial instability and require surgical stabilization.

Laxity of the transverse atlantal ligament is common in patients with Down's syndrome, with a reported incidence of 15% [12] (Fig. 1.4). The lesion may be found in all age groups, without any age preponderance [12]. These patients rupture or attenuate the transverse atlantal ligament, with encroachment of the "safe zone of steel," but at least initially are protected from spinal cord compression by the "check-rein" of the alar ligaments. In other words, many have excessive motion, but relatively few are symptomatic. The majority are discovered only by radiological survey. If radiographs of the upper cervical spine indicate an atlantal-dens interval of more than 4.5 mm, instability is considered to be present. Usually, if symptoms are present, instability of greater than 7 mm or even 10 mm is found. Recent reports suggest an increased incidence of occiput-C1 instability also.

We still know very little about the natural history of atlanto-axial instability in Down's syndrome despite the radiographic examination of hundreds of children. Some studies have suggested that some children become looser with time; others that those with small degrees of instability can, on occasion, become stable [12]. Currently, routine radiographic examination for children with Down's syndrome is recommended only if they plan to compete in athletics. Any Down's affected child with a musculoskeletal complaint such as subluxating patellae, dislocating hips, or a wide-based ataxic gait should be investigated. Similarly, if a child with Down's syndrome needs a general anesthetic, cervical spine stability should be evaluated because head and neck positioning during the procedure could lead to neurological injury. With our present knowledge, prophylactic stabilization does not appear to be indicated.

Those with a minor degree of hypermobility or instability should be followed regularly with flexion–extension radiographs. They should not engage in contact sports, somersaults, trampoline exercises, or other activities which encourage neck flexion and the potential risks should be discussed with the parents. Any child who has persisting neck symptoms caused by instability or a history of neurological problems should have surgical stabilization [12].

Odontoid Anomalies

The anomalies of the odontoid range from aplasia and hypoplasia to os odontoideum. A congenital or developmental etiology has always been assumed. Hypoplasia and os odontoideum can be acquired secondary to trauma or, rarely, infection [13]. This has led to the suggestion that some cases of os odontoideum or hypoplasia follow an unrecognized fracture of the base or damage to the epiphyseal plate of the odontoid in the first few years of life [13]. The insult could compromise the developing dens blood supply, resulting in partial failure, complete absorption, or an os odontoideum. Sankar et al. [14] support the concept that both trauma and congenital deficiency may be etiologically responsible. It is important to recognize that children who have syndromes which involve the cervical spine such as spondyloepiphyseal dysplasia or Down's syndrome, may develop os odontoideum without a history of previous trauma.

Clinical Features

Odontoid hypoplasia and os odontoideum present with similar clinical findings, caused by instability and displacement of the atlas on the axis. Patients usually present in young adult life and problems are rare in infancy [13], although we have seen cases in children under 3 years.

Congenital odontoid anomalies may be incidental findings in patients who have neck radiographs taken after trauma. This trauma may initiate the atlanto-axial instability or precipitate symptoms in an already compromised, previously asymptomatic joint. Patients may present with no symptoms (incidental diagnosis), local neck symptoms (neck pain, torticollis, and headache), transitory paresis after trauma, or myelopathy (cord compression). Neurological manifestations are recognized with increasing frequency. Although accurate statistics are not available, it is believed that more than 50% of patients either have or will develop neurological problems. These are varied: weakness and loss of balance are common complaints. Upper motor neurone signs, proprioceptive and sphincter disturbances are relatively common. Children with odontoid aplasia and an altered vertebral circulation may suffer a stroke [15].

Imaging

Odontoid aplasia is extremely rare. It is best seen in the open-mouth view. The diagnostic feature is the absence of the basilar portion of the odontoid, which normally dips down into and contributes to the body of the axis. The most common form of hypoplasia presents with a short, stubby peg of odontoid projecting just above the lateral facet articulations. Matsui et al. [16] found that the "round type," which appears to be a very flat C2, has more instability and a greater risk of severe myelopathy. This often causes a Brown-Sequard lesion suggesting a more lateral instability by comparison with the blunt stubby or "cone-shaped" os odontoideum. Watanabe et al. [17] developed an instability index to help evaluate children with an os odontoideum. They defined it as the percentage change in the space available for the cord from neck flexion to extension. Watanabe noted that children with a sagittal plane rotation angle of over 20° or an instability index of more than 40% are likely to have spinal cord signs.

However, the instability associated with os odontoideum is often multidirectional and lateral instability is more likely to cause a neurological problem [16].

Os odontoideum may be overlooked if tomograms or CT are not taken (Fig. 1.5). It appears as a radiolucent oval or round ossicle with a smooth, dense bone border. The size varies but it is usually located in the position of the normal odontoid tip or near the basioccipital bone where it may fuse with the clivus. The dens base is almost invariably hypoplastic.

It may be difficult to differentiate an os odontoideum from non-union after an odontoid fracture. With odontoid non-union, a narrow line separates the odontoid at its base. This may have either irregular or smooth edges of variable cortical thickness. The preservation of the normal shape and size of the dens on the anteroposterior view is an important distinguishing feature. Fagan et al. [18] observed that the C1 anterior arch was intimately related to the os odontoideum in a pattern they termed the "jigsaw sign". The surface interdigitation and narrowed cartilage space suggested a congenital rather than posttraumatic etiology. With os odontoideum, the gap between the os and the hypoplastic dens is wide and usually lies well above the level of the superior articular facets of the axis. The os generally does not preserve the normal shape or size of the odontoid, usually being half the size, rounded or oval, and having a smooth uniform cortex. If the os is in the area of the foramen magnum, there is little diagnostic problem.

The free ossicle of the os odontoideum usually appears fixed to the anterior arch of the atlas and moves with it in flexion and extension. The C1–C2 articulation is usually most unstable in flexion, less often so in extension, and only occasionally unstable in all directions [13]. In one series of patients, the average displacement of those undergoing surgical stabilization was 1.1 cm [13].

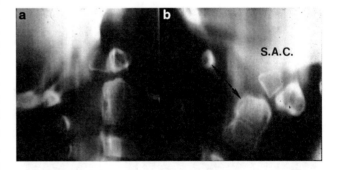

Fig. 1.5 Lateral flexion–extension radiograph of an os odontoideum: (**a**) extension; (**b**) flexion. The odontoid ossicle is fixed to the anterior ring of the atlas and moves with it in flexion and extension and lateral slide. The space available for the spinal cord (SAC) decreases with flexion and the ossicle moves into the spinal canal with extension. From Fielding et al. [13], used with permission

Treatment

Patients with congenital anomalies of the odontoid lead a precarious existence. A trivial insult superimposed on an already weakened and compromised structure may be catastrophic.

Patients with local symptoms or transient myelopathy may expect recovery, at least temporarily. Surgical stabilization is indicated for:

1. neurological involvement (even if transient);
2. instability of 10 mm or greater in flexion and extension;
3. progressive instability;
4. persistent neck complaints associated with instability.

Controversy exists as to the role of prophylactic stabilization in the asymptomatic patient with instability [13]. The possible complications of surgery must be weighed against the dangers of instability with secondary spinal cord pressure. In the paediatric age group, it may be difficult or impossible to curtail activity, even when instability is marked [13]. When fusion is undertaken, regardless of the indication, preoperative halo traction is often required to achieve reduction. This may need to be retained during surgery and postoperatively until converted to a suitable immobilization device [13].

Generally, a posterior approach is sufficient for atlanto-axial arthrodesis by the Gallie technique [19] (Fig. 1.6). When there are associated bony anomalies at the occipito-cervical junction, the fusion may need extension to the occiput. Koop et al. [20] have reported excellent results with stabilization, using a technique of flapping the occipital periosteum to the ring of C1, and external stabilization. Posterior fusion using wiring techniques and/or transarticular screw fixation may avoid the need for postoperative

halo immobilization. C1–2 transarticular screws are the first choice whenever possible [21] (Fig. 1.7). They demonstrate resistance to all three planes of movement. In adults, this construct has provided excellent outcomes and C1–2 transarticular screws have been successful in a large number of children and adolescents. However C1–2 transarticular screws cannot always be used. In 7–22% of patients, the variable location of the foramen transversarium and vulnerability of the vertebral artery make them unsafe [21–24]. The alternatives, which have been less well studied, are C1 lateral mass screws and C2 pars screws combined in a rod-cantilever construct, "the Harms construct" [21].

For irreducible deformity, anterior decompression in conjunction with posterior C1–C2 or occipito-cervical fusion, coupled with internal fixation, has given satisfactory results [25]. Patients with an os odontoideum without neurological deficit and no instability at C1–C2 can be managed without operative intervention. Nonetheless, in these patients, longitudinal clinical and radiographic surveillance is recommended [25].

Klippel–Feil Syndrome

Congenital cervical fusion is the result of failure of the normal segmentation of the cervical somites during the third to eighth weeks of life. With the exception of a few patients in whom this condition is inherited, the etiology is as yet undetermined. It is important to note that the effect of this embryological abnormality is not limited to the cervical spine. Patients with the Klippel–Feil syndrome, even those with minor cervical lesions, may have defects in the genitourinary, nervous, and cardiopulmonary systems, and even hearing impairment [26]. Many of these "hidden" abnormalities may be more detrimental to the patient's general well-being than the obvious deformity in the neck.

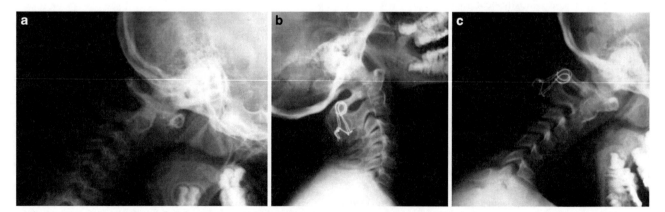

Fig. 1.6 This 7-year-old had a 1-year history of peculiar posturing and stiffness of the neck. (**a**) Flexion and (**b**) Extension and (**c**) flexion radiographs taken after posterior stabilization. Reduction must be accomplished before surgery, and if wire stabilization is selected, care must be taken to avoid further flexion of the neck during passage of the wire under C1

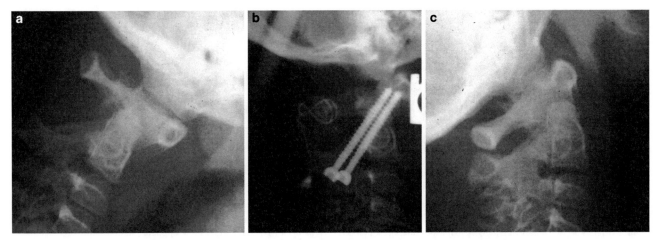

Fig. 1.7 An 8-year-old with Down's syndrome with C1–C2 instability secondary to os odontoideum. (**a**) Flexion view demonstrates instability with significant compromise in the space available for the spinal cord. (**c**) Extension view demonstrates that the C1 ring reduces satisfactorily with C2. (**b**) Postoperative view demonstrates transarticular screws and posterior wire fixation of C1–C2. The patient fused quickly, is asymptomatic, and fully active

In the review by Hensinger et al. [26], a high incidence of related congenital anomalies was reported, emphasizing that all patients with the Klippel–Feil syndrome should be thoroughly investigated.

Symptoms

With the exception of the anomalies that involve the atlanto-axial joint, there are no symptoms that can be directly attributed to the fused cervical vertebrae. All symptoms commonly associated with the Klippel–Feil syndrome originate at the open segments, where the remaining free articulations may show compensatory hypermobility. Symptoms may then arise from two sources:

1. Mechanical symptoms caused by irritation of the joints.
2. Neurological symptoms caused by root irritation or spinal cord compression.

The majority of patients who develop symptoms are in the second or third decade of life, suggesting that the instability is in part a function of time, with increasing ligament laxity.

Clinical Features

The classical clinical description of the syndrome is a triad of low posterior hairline, short neck, and limitation of neck motion (Figs. 1.8a, b), but fewer than 50% of the patients have all three signs. Clinically, the most consistent finding is limitation of neck movement. Shortening of the neck, unless extreme, is a subtle finding. Similarly, the low posterior hairline is not constant. Fewer than 20% of patients with the Klippel–Feil syndrome have obvious facial asymmetry, torticollis, or webbing of the neck.

Sprengel's deformity (Chapter 2 of Children's Upper and Lower Limb Orthopaedic Disorders) occurs in 17–33% of patients [27]. Other clinical features are occasionally found: ptosis of the eye, Duane's contracture (contracture of the lateral rectus muscle), lateral rectus palsy, facial nerve palsy, and a cleft or high arched palate. Abnormalities of the upper extremities include syndactyly, thumb hypoplasia, supernumerary digits, and hypoplasia of the upper extremity. Abnormalities of the lower extremities are infrequent [26].

Imaging Features

In the severely affected child, adequate radiographic evaluation can be difficult. Fixed bony deformities frequently prevent proper positioning, and overlapping shadows from the mandible, occiput, or foramen magnum may obscure the upper vertebrae. CT scanning coupled with flexion–extension radiographs of the cervical spine (Figs. 1.8c, d) can delineate more precisely the presence or absence of spinal cord compression. MRI is also useful. Apart from vertebral fusion, flattening and widening of the involved vertebral bodies and absent disc spaces are the most common findings (Figs. 1.9 and 1.10).

Narrowing of the spinal canal, if it occurs, usually manifests in adult life and is due to degenerative changes (osteoarthritic spurs) or hypermobility. Enlargement of the cervical canal is uncommon and, if found, may

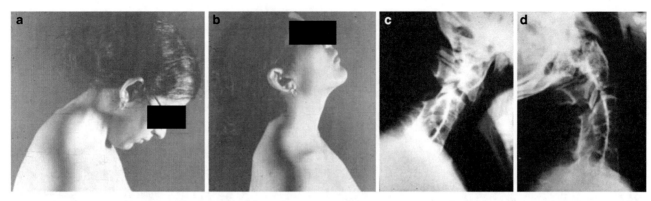

Fig. 1.8 An 18-year-old female with the Klippel–Feil syndrome demonstrating flexion–extension of the cervical spine, both clinically (**a** and **b**) and radiologically (**c** and **d**). The majority of the neck motion is occurring at the C3–C4 disc space. Clinically, the patient is able to maintain adequate range (90°) of flexion–extension. At the time of these examinations, she was asymptomatic, but with aging this hypermobile articulation may become unstable. This article was published in: Hensinger RN, MacEwen GD. Congenital abnormalities of the spine. In: Rothman RH, Simeone FA, eds. The Spine. Philadelphia: Elsevier; 1982:219. Copyright Elsevier; 1982

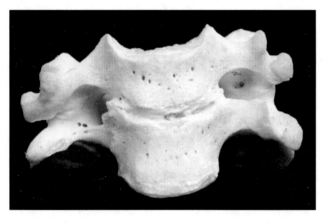

Fig. 1.9 Anterior view of a postmortem specimen of a congenital block vertebra of C3–C4. The specimen demonstrates complete fusion, but remnants of the cartilaginous vertebral endplates can still be seen

Associated Conditions

Scoliosis/Kyphosis

Scoliosis is the most frequent anomaly found in association with the syndrome [26], with 60% of patients having a significant curve.

Renal Abnormalities

In the Klippel–Feil syndrome, more than 33% of the children can be expected to have a significant urinary tract anomaly, which is often asymptomatic in the young.

Sprengel's Deformity

Sprengel's deformity occurs in 17–33% of Klippel–Feil patients. There is no specific correlation with fusion patterns, gender, the number of fused segments, or the degree of cervical scoliosis [27].

Cardiovascular Abnormalities

Up to 14% of patients have congenital heart disease.

Deafness

The otology literature has reported hearing impairment and deafness in more than 30% of patients with Klippel–Feil syndrome. Other defects include absence of the auditory canal

indicate the presence of conditions such as a syringomyelia, hydromyelia, or the Arnold–Chiari malformation.

All these defects may extend into the upper thoracic spine, particularly in the severely affected patient. A disturbance of the upper thoracic spine on a routine chest radiograph may be the first clue to an unrecognized cervical synostosis. When a high thoracic congenital scoliosis is being assessed, the radiographic evaluation should routinely include lateral flexion–extension views of the cervical spine. In a group of 33 patients with the Klippel–Feil syndrome, occipitalization occurred in nearly half and fusion in the C2–C3 segment was noted in 72% [7]. When these are combined, there is a great propensity for instability at the atlanto-axial joint. However, the authors found that minor degrees of hypermobility at the atlanto-axial junction were not necessarily associated with an increased risk of symptoms or neurological signs.

Fig. 1.10 (**a**) Radiographs of a 7-year-old demonstrating posterior fusion of the laminae and spinous process, but incomplete fusion of the vertebral bodies anteriorly. (**b**) Same patient at age 20 years, now demonstrating complete fusion of the vertebral bodies C1–C2 and C3–C7. In children, narrowing of the cervical disc spaces cannot always be appreciated, as ossification of vertebral bodies is not completed until adolescence. The unossified cartilage endplates can give a false impression of a normal disc space

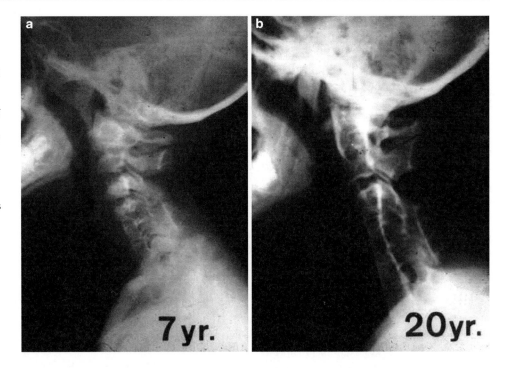

and microtia. There is no characteristic audiological anomaly and all types of hearing loss have been described.

Mirror Motions (Synkinesia)

Synkinesia consists of involuntary paired movements of the hands and, occasionally, the arms. It was first described by Bauman [28], who found it to be present in four of six patients with the Klippel–Feil syndrome. Approximately 20% demonstrate mirror motions clinically [26].

Treatment

The minimally affected patient with the Klippel–Feil syndrome can be expected to lead a normal active life, with no or only minor restrictions. Many severely affected patients will enjoy the same good prognosis if early and appropriate treatment is instituted when needed. This is particularly applicable in the area of associated Sprengel's deformity, scoliosis, and renal abnormalities. Prevention of further deformity or complications can be of great benefit to the patient. Those patients with major areas of cervical synostosis or high-risk patterns of cervical spine motion should be strongly advised to avoid activities that place stress on the cervical spine. Theiss et al. [29] found that 22% of the patients with the Klippel–Feil syndrome and congenital scoliosis developed cervical symptoms on long-term follow-up. Some fusion patterns put them at particular risk. There was a greater

likelihood of neck symptoms with fusion at the cervico-thoracic junction and congenital cervical stenosis. Pizzutillo et al. [30] reported on long-term follow-up that individuals with Klippel–Feil syndrome who had hypermobility of the upper cervical segments were at risk of neurological sequelae. Those with alteration in motion in the lower cervical segment were more likely to develop degenerative disease. Sudden neurological compromise or death after minor trauma has been reported in the Klippel–Feil syndrome and is usually the result of disruption at the hypermobile articulation. The role of prophylactic surgical stabilization in the asymptomatic patient has not yet been defined.

Differential Diagnosis of Torticollis

Torticollis, or wry-neck, is a common childhood complaint. The etiology is diverse and identifying the cause can be difficult.

Congenital muscular torticollis is the most common cause in the infant and young child, but there are other problems that lead to this unusual posture. Head tilt and rotatory deformity of the head and neck (torticollis) usually indicate a problem at C1–C2, whereas head tilt alone indicates a more generalized problem in the cervical spine. If the posturing of the head and neck is noted at or shortly after birth, congenital anomalies of the cervical spine, particularly those that involve C1–C2, typically present as a rigid deformity, and the sternocleidomastoid muscle is not contracted or in spasm.

Approximately 20% of patients with the Klippel–Feil syndrome have associated torticollis [26, 31]. With asymmetric development of the occipital condyles or the facets of C1, the head tilt may result in a torticollis unless compensated for by a tilt of the lower cervical spine such as occurs in the milder forms [11].

Inflammatory conditions such as cervical lymphadenitis may cause a wry-neck tilt. A less frequent cause is a retropharyngeal abscess complicating posterior pharyngeal inflammation or tonsillitis. Children with polyarticular juvenile idiopathic arthritis often develop cervical joint involvement: torticollis and limited neck movement may be the only clinical signs. Spontaneous atlanto-axial rotatory subluxation may follow acute pharyngitis [31]. A rare inflammatory cause is acute calcification of a cervical disc, which can be seen on plain radiographs.

Trauma should always be considered and carefully excluded. If unrecognized it may have serious neurological consequences. In general, torticollis most commonly follows injury to the Cl–C2 articulation. Minor trauma can lead to spontaneous C1–C2 subluxation. Fracture or dislocation of the odontoid may not be apparent on the initial radiographs and, consequently, a high index of suspicion and careful follow-up are required.

Children with bone dysplasia, Morquio's syndrome, spondyloepiphyseal dysplasia, and Down's syndrome have a high incidence of Cl–C2 instability and should be evaluated routinely.

Intermittent torticollis can occur in the young child. A seizure-like disorder called benign paroxysmal torticollis of infancy is due to many neurological causes, including drug intoxication. Similarly, Sandifer's syndrome, involving gastro-esophageal reflux with sudden posturing of the trunk and torticollis, is being recognized more often, particularly in the neurologically handicapped child, for example, with cerebral palsy [32].

Neurological disorders, particularly space-occupying lesions of the central nervous system, such as tumors of the posterior fossa or spinal column, chordoma and syringomyelia, are often accompanied by torticollis. Generally, there will be additional neurological findings such as long-tract signs and weakness in the upper extremities. Uncommon neurological causes include dystonia musculorum deformans and problems of hearing and vision that can result in head tilt. Although uncommon, hysterical and psychogenic causes exist, but should be diagnosed only after other causes have been excluded.

Radiographs

All children with torticollis should be evaluated with radiographs to exclude a bony abnormality or fracture.

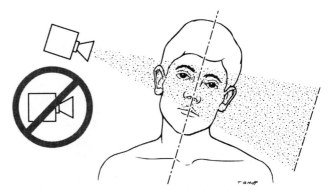

Ring of C1 stays with the Occiput

Fig. 1.11 Obtaining a satisfactory radiograph may be hampered by the patient's limited ability to cooperate, fixed bony deformity, and overlapping shadows from the mandible, occiput and foramen magnum. A helpful guide is that the atlas moves with the occiput, and if the X-ray beam is directed 90° to the lateral of the skull, a satisfactory view of the occipito-cervical junction usually results

Radiographic interpretation of congenital torticollis may be difficult because of the fixed abnormal head position and restricted motion. In those with a painful wry-neck, it may be impossible to position the child appropriately for a standard view of the occipito-cervical junction. A helpful guide is that the atlas moves with the occiput, so that if the X-ray beam is directed 90° to the lateral skull, a satisfactory view of the occipito-cervical junction is usually obtained (Fig. 1.11). Flexion–extension stress films, laminograms, or cineradiography may be necessary to confirm atlanto-axial instability.

Atlanto-Axial Rotary Displacement

The onset of the problem may be spontaneous, associated with trivial trauma, or may follow an upper respiratory tract infection. Typically, the child awakes with a "crick" in the neck and, with little or no treatment, this resolves within 1 week. Rarely, these deformities persist and the child presents with a resistant, unresolving torticollis, best described as atlanto-axial rotary fixation or fixed atlanto-axial displacement.

This problem can occur within the normal range of motion or with anterior shift of the atlas on the axis as a result of fractures of C1 and C2 or ligamentous deficiency, leading to atlanto-axial instability. Neurological deficits may rarely be associated with rotary displacements, particularly with anterior displacement.

The etiology of this type of displacement remains theoretical, because insufficient anatomical and postmortem evidence is available. The obstruction is probably capsular and synovial interposition, which produces pain in the

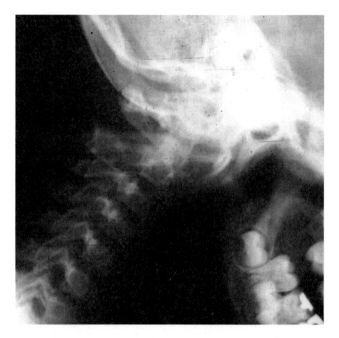

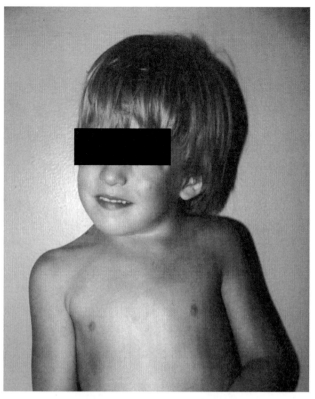

Fig. 1.12 Marked anterior displacement of C1 on C2 found in a patient with atlanto-axial rotatory fixation of 2 months' duration

initial stages, with resultant muscle spasm. The spasm holds the neck in flexion and may aggravate forward displacement of C1 on C2 (Fig. 1.12).

Fig. 1.13 Typical torticollis position of atlanto-axial rotatory displacement (cock robin), with the head rotated in one direction and tilted to the opposite side, with slight flexion

Clinical Features

The torticollis position is likened to a robin listening for a worm or the "cocked robin" position (Fig. 1.13). The head is tilted to one side and rotated to the opposite side, with slight flexion. When the condition is acute, the child resists attempts to move the head, complaining of marked pain with any passive attempts to do so. Associated muscle spasm, unlike muscular torticollis, is predominantly on the side of the "long" sternocleidomastoid, because this muscle is attempting to correct the deformity. If the deformity becomes fixed, the pain will subside but the torticollis will persist, associated with a diminished range of neck motion. In long-standing cases, particularly in younger children, facial asymmetry with flattening may develop.

Imaging Features

In the acute stages, the diagnosis depends primarily on history and clinical evidence, because plain radiographs are not diagnostic. In the open-mouth anteroposterior and lateral projections, the lateral mass of C1 that has rotated forward

appears wider and closer to the midline (medial offset), whereas the opposite lateral mass is narrower and away from the midline (lateral offset). One of the facet joints may be obscured because of apparent overlapping.

On the lateral projection, the wedge-shaped lateral mass of the atlas lies anteriorly, where the oval arch of the atlas normally lies. The posterior arches of the atlas fail to superimpose because of head tilt. This may suggest assimilation of the atlas to the occiput because head tilt allows the skull to obscure C1. Flexion–extension stress films rule out the anterior displacement of atlas on axis that is occasionally seen with rotary displacement.

Type I rotary displacement is by far the most common form seen in children (Fig. 1.14). It is more benign and may be managed expectantly. The type II deformity is potentially more dangerous needs carefully management. Type III and IV deformities are rare, but neurological involvement or even instant death may follow and demand very careful treatment. CT has largely replaced cineradiology as the radiological technique of choice for this condition (Fig. 1.15). In children with suspected atlanto-axial rotary displacement, Been et al. [33] recommend CT scanning under general anesthesia. Patients improve if the examination is normal.

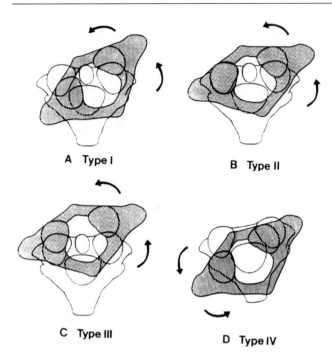

A   Type I   B   Type II

C   Type III   D   Type IV

Fig. 1.14 Classification of rotatory displacement. From Fielding and Hawkins [31], used with permission

Treatment

Many cases of atlanto-axial rotary displacement prove transitory. The stiff neck and slightly twisted head resolve in a few days. If the complaints are mild and have been present for less than 1 week, we advise a simple soft collar and analgesics. If there is no spontaneous improvement or the symptoms persist, more aggressive treatment should be instituted. When simple measures fail, we suggest bed rest, halter

traction, muscle relaxants, and analgesics. If the atlas is displaced anteriorly on the axis, gradual reduction should be obtained, followed by immobilization in the corrected position in a Minerva cast for 6 weeks to allow ligamentous healing. Careful follow-up is necessary because of the potential for continued atlanto-axial instability.

If the condition has been present for 1–3 months, halo traction is often necessary to achieve reduction. However, the C1–C2 articulation may not stabilize after immobilization and then needs surgical correction and fusion. If the condition has been present for over 3 months, the deformity typically is fixed. In those whose spinal canal is compromised by anterior C1 displacement, a further insult could be catastrophic. C1–C2 fusion is indicated to achieve stability and to maintain correction.

Congenital Muscular Torticollis (Congenital Wry-Neck)

Torticollis is common in the first 6–8 weeks of life. The deformity is caused by contracture of the sternocleido-mastoid muscle, with the head tilted toward the involved side and the chin rotated toward the contralateral shoulder (Fig. 1.16). If the infant is examined within the first 4 weeks of life, a mass or "tumor" is usually palpable in the neck (Fig. 1.17). It is generally a non-tender, soft enlargement that is mobile beneath the skin and attached to or located within the body of the sternocleidomastoid. The mass attains maximum size within the first 1 month of life and then gradually regresses. If the child is examined after 4–6 months of age, the mass is usually absent, and contracture of the

Fig. 1.15 Dynamic CT scan of the upper cervical spine in atlanto-axial rotatory subluxation. (**a**) The head is rotated approximately 45° to one side, with the contralateral lateral mass of C1 moving forward on the facet of C2. (**b**) The head cannot be rotated past the midline, and the relationship of C1–C2 is unchanged. From Phillips WA, Hensinger RN. The management of rotatory atlanto-axial subluxation in children. J Bone Joint Surg 1989; 71A:665. Used with permission

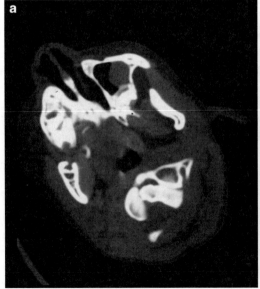
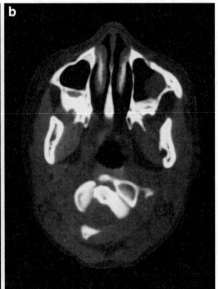

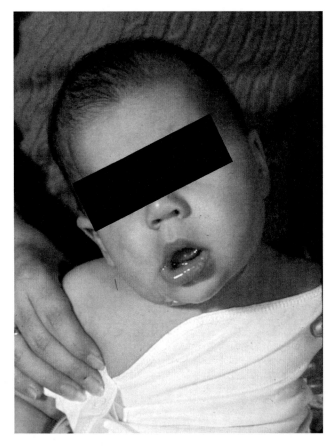

Fig. 1.16 A 6-month-old infant with right-sided congenital muscular torticollis. Note the rotation of the skull and asymmetry and flattening of the face on the side of the contracted sternocleidomastoid

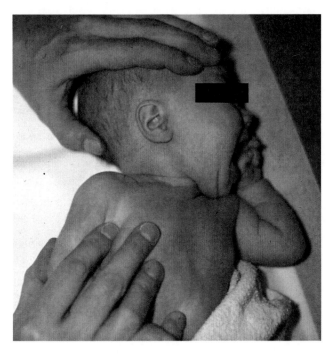

Fig. 1.17 Six-week-old infant with swelling in the region of the sternocleidomastoid muscle. The mass is usually soft, non-tender, and mobile beneath the skin, but is attached to the muscle

sternocleidomastoid muscle and the torticollis posture are the only clinical findings (Fig. 1.16).

If the condition is progressive, deformities of the face and skull can result, and they are usually apparent within the first year. Flattening of the face on the side of the contracted sternocleidomastoid muscle may be marked (Fig. 1.16). If the condition remains untreated during the growth years, the level of the eyes and ears becomes distorted and may result in considerable cosmetic deformity.

Etiology

Birth records of affected children demonstrate a preponderance of breech or difficult deliveries or primiparous births [34]. However, the deformity may occur with normal delivery and in infants born by Cesarean section [34]. In one study, half the patients had a difficult delivery, 7% were born by Cesarean section and 44% by uncomplicated vaginal delivery [35]. Difficult deliveries included breech presentation, vacuum extraction and forceps instrumentation. Microscopic examination of resected surgical specimens and experimental work suggest that the lesion is caused by occlusion of the venous outflow of the sternocleidomastoid muscle. This leads to edema, muscle fiber degeneration and eventually, fibrosis. The problem may be caused by uterine crowding or "packing" because in 75% of children in one study the lesion was right sided [34]. In addition, 20% of children with congenital muscular torticollis have congenital dysplasia of the hip, similarly associated with restricted infant movement in the tight maternal space. In a more recent publication, 6% of children with developmental dysplasia of the hip (DDH) were diagnosed subsequently with congenital muscular torticollis [35]. Infants less than 1 month at diagnosis were at greater risk (9%) and boys were at greater risk of having both conditions.

Imaging

It is probably unnecessary to take radiographs of all neonates with a typical sternomastoid tumor. Radiographs of the cervical spine should be taken to exclude bony anomaly if infants fail to respond to simple stretching or if the torticollis, is atypical. Tatli et al. [36] found cervical ultrasound to be helpful in the diagnosis of congenital torticollis, identifying a fusiform enlargement of the muscle. They identified two clinical groups, one with (85%) and one without (15%) the swelling. In considering a compartment syndrome, MRI was inconsistent, did not alter treatment, and is not therefore recommended in assessment [37].

Treatment

Conservative

Most respond to a range of motion exercises supervised by a physiotherapist and carried out by the family [34, 38]. Ninety-five percent of children treated at a mean age of 2.3 months resolved with early aggressive treatment [36]. If treatment begins before 6 weeks and the infant has no neck mass, the prognosis is excellent. If the neck mass persists for more than 6 weeks, persistent deformity may follow [36].

Additional treatment measures include positioning the crib and toys so that the neck will be stretched when the infant reaches and grasps. Using a "sleeping helmet" to reduce deformity and hasten face and skull remodeling [39] is rarely necessary.

Operation

If the condition persists beyond 1 year, non-operative measures rarely succeed [38]. Similarly, established facial asymmetry and movement limited by more than 10° usually preclude a good result and operation is needed to prevent further facial flattening and poor cosmesis [38]. However, a good (but not perfect) cosmetic result may be obtained as late as 12 years of age. Asymmetry of the skull and face will improve as long as adequate growth potential remains once the deforming pull of the sternocleidomastoid is removed.

The operation should completely section the distal insertion of the sternocleidomastoid muscle. It is important to release fascial bands. In the older child it may be necessary to divide the muscle proximally at its mastoid origin in addition. Recently, endoscopic release has been used to reduce scarring and the risk of injuring the spinal accessory nerve or greater auricular nerve [40]. The entire muscle should not be excised, because this may lead to reverse torticollis [34] or additional deformity. The postoperative regimen includes passive stretching exercises in the same manner as those performed preoperatively. The night use of halter traction at home may help. Bracing or cast correction may be necessary if the deformity is long-standing. The results of surgery are uniformly good with a low incidence of complications or recurrence [34, 38]. If the patient is young, the facial asymmetry can be expected to resolve completely [34].

References

1. Klippel M, Feil A. Un cas d'absence des vertebras cervicales avec cage thoracique. remontant jusqu'à la base du crane. Nouvelle Iconographie de la Salpetrière. 1912; 25:223–250.
2. McRae DL. The significance of abnormalities of the cervical spine. Am J Roentgenol 1960; 84:3–25.
3. Erbengi A, Oge HK. Congenital malformations of the cranioverte-bral junction: classification and surgical treatment. Acta Neurochir (Wien) 1994; 127:180–185.
4. Chamberlain WE. Basilar impression (platybasia): bizarre developmental anatomy of occipital bone and upper cervical spine with striking and misleading neurologic manifestation. Yale J Biol Med 1939; 11:487–496.
5. McGregor M. The significance of certain measurements of the skull in the diagnosis of basilar impression. Br J Radiol 1948; 21:171–181.
6. Gholve PA, Hosalkar HS, Ricchetti ET, et al. Occipitalization of the atlas in children. Morphologic classification, associations, and clinical relevance. J Bone Joint Surg Am 2007; 89:571–578.
7. Shen FH, Samartzis D, Herman J, et al. Radiographic assessment of segmental motion at the atlantoaxial junction in the Klippel-Feil patient. Spine 2006; 31:171–177.
8. Rouvreau P, Glorion, C, Langlais, J, et al. Assessment and neurologic involvement of patients with cervical spine congenital synostosis as in Klippel–Feil syndrome: study of 19 cases. J Pediatr Orthop 1998; 7B:179–185.
9. Samartzis D, Kalluri P, Herman J, et al. Superior odontoid migration in the Klippel-Feil patient. Eur Spine J 2007; 16:1489–1497.
10. Senoglu M, Safavi-Abbasi S, Theodore N, et al. The frequency and clinical significance of congenital defects of the posterior and anterior arch of the atlas. J Neurosurg Spine 2007; 7:399–402.
11. Dubousset J. Torticollis in children caused by congenital anomalies of the atlas. J Bone Joint Surg Am 1986; 68:178–188.
12. Burke SW, French HG, Roberts JM, et al. Chronic atlanto-axial instability in Down syndrome. J Bone Joint Surg Am 1985; 67:1356–1360.
13. Fielding JW, Hensinger RN, Hawkins RJ. Os odontoideum. J Bone Joint Surg Am 1980; 62:376–383.
14. Sankar WN, Wills BP, Dormans JP, et al. Os odontoideum revisited: the case for a multifactorial etiology. Spine 2006; 31:979–984.
15. Phillips PC, Lorentsen KJ, Shropshire LC, et al. Congenital odontoid aplasia and posterior circulation stroke in childhood. Ann Neurol 1988; 23:410–413.
16. Matsui H, Imada K, Tsuji H. Radiographic classification of Os odontoideum and its clinical significance. Spine 1997; 22:1706–1709.
17. Watanabe M, Toyama Y, Fujimura Y. Atlantoaxial instability in os odontoideum with myelopathy. Spine 1996; 21:1435–1439.
18. Fagan AB, Askin GN, Earwaker JW. The jigsaw sign. A reliable indicator of congenital aetiology in os odontoideum. Eur Spine J 2004; 13:295–300.
19. Stabler CL, Eismont FJ, Brown MD, et al. Failure of posterior cervical fusions using cadaveric bone graft in children. J Bone Joint Surg Am 1985; 67:371–375.
20. Koop SE, Winter RB, Lonstein JE. The surgical treatment of instability of the upper part of the cervical spine in children and adolescents. J Bone Joint Surg Am 1984; 66:403–411.
21. Anderson RC, Ragel BT, Mocco J, et al. Selection of a rigid internal fixation construct for stabilization at the craniovertebral junction in pediatric patients. J Neurosurg 2007; 107:36–42.
22. Brockmeyer DL, York JE, Apfelbaum RI. Anatomical suitability of C1–2 transarticular screw placement in pediatric patients. J Neurosurg 2000; 92:7–11.
23. Igarashi T, Kikuchi S, Sato K, et al. Anatomic study of the axis for surgical planning of transarticular screw fixation. Clin Orthop Rel Res 2003; 408:162–166.
24. Madawi AA, Casey AT, Solanki GA, et al. Radiological and anatomical evaluation of the atlantoaxial transarticular screw fixation technique. J Neurosurg 1997; 86:961–968.

25. Os odontoideum. Neurosurgery 2002; 50:S148–155.
26. Hensinger RN, Lang JE, MacEwen GD. Klippel–Feil syndrome; a constellation of associated anomalies. J Bone Joint Surg Am 1974; 56:1246–1253.
27. Samartzis D, Herman J, Lubicky JP, et al. Sprengel's deformity in Klippel–Feil syndrome. Spine 2007; 32:E512–516.
28. Bauman G. Absence of the cervical spine: Klippel–Feil syndrome. JAMA 1998; 98:129–132.
29. Theiss SM, Smith MD, Winter RB. The long-term follow-up of patients with Klippel–Feil syndrome and congenital scoliosis. Spine 1997; 22:1219–1222.
30. Pizzutillo PD, Woods M, Nicholson L, et al. Risk factors in Klippel–Feil syndrome. Spine 1994; 19:2110–2116.
31. Fielding JW, Hawkins RJ. Atlanto-axial rotatory fixation. (Fixed rotatory subluxation of the atlanto-axial joint). J Bone Joint Surg Am 1977; 59:37–44.
32. Sutcliff J. Torsion spasms and abnormal postures in children with hiatus hernia: Sandifer's syndrome. Prog Pediatr Radiol 1969; 2:190–197.
33. Been HD, Kerkhoffs GM, Maas M. Suspected atlantoaxial rotatory fixation-subluxation: the value of multidetector computed tomography scanning under general anesthesia. Spine 2007; 32:E163–167.
34. MacDonald D. Sternomastoid tumour and muscular torticollis. J Bone Joint Surg Br 1969; 51:432–443.
35 von Heideken J, Green DW, Burke SW, et al. The relationship between developmental dysplasia of the hip and congenital muscular torticollis. J Pediatr Orthop 2006; 26:805–808.
36 Tatli B, Aydinli N, Caliskan M, et al. Congenital muscular torticollis: evaluation and classification. Pediatr Neurol 2006; 34:41–44.
37. Parikh SN, Crawford AH, Choudhury S. Magnetic resonance imaging in the evaluation of infantile torticollis. Orthopedics 2004; 27:509–515.
38. Canale ST, Griffin DW, Hubbard CN. Congenital muscular torticollis. A long-term follow-up. J Bone Joint Surg Am 1982; 64:810–816.
39. Clarren SK, Smith DW, Hanson JW. Helmet treatment for plagiocephaly and congenital muscular torticollis. J Pediatr 1979; 94:43–46.
40. Swain B. Transaxillary endoscopic release of restricting bands in congenital muscular torticollis—a novel technique. J Plast Reconstr Aesthet Surg 2007; 60:95–98.

Chapter 2

Back Pain in Children

Robert A. Dickson

Introduction

Back pain in childhood, while uncommon, is often associated with serious underlying pathology. In one series of 210 cases [1], infection or neoplasia proved to be the underlying cause in more than 40% of patients younger than 12 years of age. After this age, there is a relative increase in non-specific causes of backache. Adolescent back pain is associated with decreased mobility of the lumbar spine and stiffness of the hip and knee joints [2]. Back pain in the adolescent age group is more common in girls and also exhibits a familial pattern [3]. During later adolescence, trauma, mechanical, and early degenerative disorders are more frequent causes of back pain, and serious pathology affects only a small proportion.

In young children, back pain tends to be vague and poorly localized. Consequently spinal or paraspinal pathology in the young may be easily missed or incorrectly diagnosed, with adverse effects upon subsequent treatment and outcome. Careful clinical evaluation, appropriate investigation, and a grasp of the likely causes for each age group minimize the likelihood of that unsatisfactory state of affairs.

Assessment of the Child

While older children and adolescents can often give a clear history of their back pain, localizing it well and describing neurological symptoms, this is not so in the infant or younger child who may just be irritable, with a stiff back and

R.A. Dickson (✉)
Academic Unit of Orthopaedic Surgery, Leeds General Infirmary, Leeds, UK

a reluctance to move or weight-bear. In this very young age group meaningful examination can be difficult, so it is best to assess the child on mother's lap in a warm quiet environment. It is often only possible to observe the presence or absence of movement of major muscle groups and, perhaps, muscle wasting since an irritable young child often prevents any further neurological examination. When assessed prone, muscle spasm, swelling, and abnormal alignment may be seen; it is very important to palpate for spinal tenderness (only present with infection or fresh injury). With infection, especially if associated with a psoas abscess, abdominal pain and tenderness are common and may mimic renal or retroperitoneal sepsis.

The older child and adolescent can be more meaningfully assessed and both kyphotic and scoliotic deformities are best visualized in the forward bending position. When a thoracic kyphosis is present, forward bending demonstrates either a smooth hyperkyphosis with postural, roundback deformity or an angular one in association with Scheuermann's disease or localized pathology.

Idiopathic scoliosis is not usually painful except for a fatigue-type discomfort over the rotational prominence. If pain is severe, particularly at night, or if there is an atypical curve pattern such as a progressive left thoracic curve in a male then underlying pathology (tumor or syrinx) must be excluded. In the case of lumbosacral pain (with or without a local step), spondylolysis, spondylolisthesis, or adolescent disc syndrome should be suspected, particularly if associated with significant lumbosacral stiffness, tight hamstrings, or neurological deficit. Ankylosing spondylitis is another, but unusual, cause of back stiffness. It is important to differentiate between spine and hip movement particularly during the composite, forward flexion of back movement.

A more adequate neurological assessment can be carried out in the older child and adolescent. Power in all muscle groups and sensation in all lower limb dermatomes should be examined along with all reflexes, including the abdominals which may be suppressed or asymmetrical in the presence of a syrinx.

Congenital Spinal Anomalies

Be wary of blaming troublesome back symptoms on a congenital malformation: it may be a coincidental finding. The various types of congenital scoliosis and kyphosis, even when associated with dysraphism, rarely cause pain unless they produce secondary mechanical effects. The child or adolescent with a painful scoliosis should be assumed, until proven otherwise, to have an underlying tumor (such as osteoid osteoma) or infection.

Spinal Trauma

In general, the paediatric spine is remarkably resistant to trauma because of its suppleness and spinal cord injuries are therefore rare. However, Kewalramani and Tori [4] found a much higher incidence of cord injury in children under 15 years of age, accounting for one-tenth of all spinal cord injuries. They also reported a preponderance of cervical injuries. In this age group about 50% suffer incomplete or complete paralysis.

Spinal cord injury without obvious radiographic abnormality (SCIWORA) is encountered frequently in the elderly, whose pre-existing degenerative neck disease and spurs of bone already indent the spinal cord and render it vulnerable to, for example, a whiplash flexion injury. It not uncommonly occurs also in children with pristine but hypermobile neck joints and is peculiar to the cervical spine. Consequently neck radiographs can be entirely normal, but physiological displacements, curvatures, and variations in ossification are the subtle features that point to the diagnosis [5].

Most children, particularly younger ones, sustain spinal trauma as a result of a road traffic accident, while older children are usually injured in a sporting mishap [4]. The upper cervical spine is greatly over-represented in children as the site of injury [6], the atlanto-axial level being notorious. A central cord pattern of spinal cord injury is usually produced. The problem is discussed in detail in Chapter 5.

In infancy back trauma raises the possibility of non-accidental injury. Cullen in 1975 demonstrated that vertebral collapse particularly in the thoraco-lumbar region can be part of the battered baby syndrome [7]. Therefore a lateral view of the thoraco-lumbar spine is recommended as part of the non-accidental injury radiograph series [8] (Fig. 2.1).

With thoraco-lumbar spinal injuries, after the initial acute pain subsides, the symptoms can persist or worsen if a traumatic kyphosis develops. There is usually some increase in kyphosis from compression of the cancellous bone of the affected vertebral body but significantly progressive kyphosis suggests a Salter type V injury to the growth plate. Eventually the pain does tend to settle but a considerable post-traumatic kyphosis may warrant surgical correction, as does severe Scheuermann's disease.

The growing spine can be traumatized iatrogenically by way of laminectomy, undertaken surgically to deal with spinal cord tumors or other problems (Fig. 2.2). The tension band function of the posterior column is lost, leading to progressive kyphosis. A combined approach from a neurosurgeon and an orthopaedic spinal surgeon, the latter instrumenting and fusing the spine after laminectomy, guards against subsequent deformity.

Spinal Infection

While spinal infection still represents a problem in the developing world, only 2–4% of infections in the developed world involve the spine [9]. Two-thirds are pyogenic and one-third

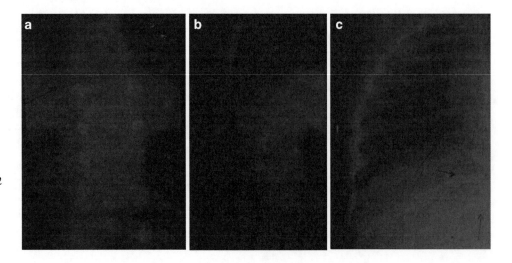

Fig. 2.1 The spine in child abuse. (**a**) Anteroposterior (AP) view showing soft tissue shadowing (*arrows*) at the T11/12 level. (**b**) Lateral radiograph showing a wedge compression fracture. (**c**) AP radiograph of right ribs showing multiple healing fractures (*arrows*)

Fig. 2.2 Post-laminectomy kyphosis in a growing child. (**a**) AP view of the lumbar spine showing a decompressive laminectomy for spinal stenosis in a 15-year-old boy with achondroplasia. (**b**) Lateral radiograph of the lumbar spine 2 years later. With loss of the posterior tension band the spine has collapsed into 90° of kyphosis. (**c**) Lateral radiograph of the lumbar spine after anterior release and interbody grafting and posterior instrumentation

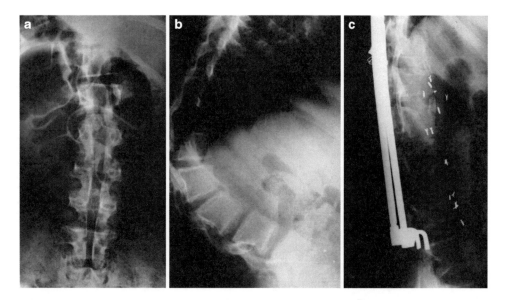

tuberculous, but the initial presentation is often very similar and in both there is commonly a delay or failure in making the correct diagnosis which leads to chronicity [10].

More than 50% of pyogenic infections are due to the *Staphylococcus aureus*, the remainder being caused by *Streptococci, Escherichia coli, Pseudomonas, Pneumococcus, Meningococcus, Salmonella, Brucella*, and fungi. With an increasing number of human immunodeficiency virus (HIV)-positive patients unusual organisms are being detected with more mixed growth patterns and increased antibiotic resistance. Previous antibiotic administration makes it difficult to isolate the offending organism. Tuberculosis is now universally caused by the human rather than the bovine bacillus.

The final common pathway for organisms tracking into the vertebra is by way of the rich vascular supply to the spine and, in particular, Batson's plexus of veins. This communicates freely with the valveless vertebral veins which spread from the occiput to the coccyx [11]. However, it is thought that the rich arterial route to the spine is probably the more important, organisms entering the vertebral bodies by the anterior and posterior nutrient foramina [12]. Here they flourish in the richly vascular metaphyseal region close to the end plate. This increased blood supply in the immature spine probably accounts for the greater prevalence of infection in the young. The relatively avascular nucleus may suffer infarction as a result of pressure from local pus or toxins and from vascular spasm. Disc resorption is particularly common in pyogenic infection as the discs are much more resistant to tuberculous infection.

As the infection gains momentum there is vertebral collapse on each side of the disc region with end plate perforation (Fig. 2.3). Abscess formation is much more obvious

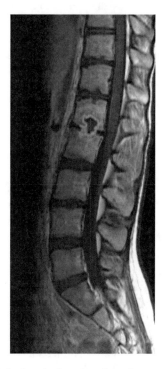

Fig. 2.3 T2-weighted sagittal section of the thoraco-lumbar spine of a teenager showing pyogenic osteomyelitis with disc space narrowing and end plate perforation

in tuberculous infection, and this can spread anteriorly in the lumbar region to the psoas muscle sheath and posteriorly into the epidural space. Compression of the spinal cord results not only from the abscess but also from locally sequestrated bone and disc fragments and an increasing kyphotic deformity. Cord compromise in tuberculosis is caused by spasm of the arterial supply, bacterial meningitis, or fibrotic constriction of the meninges.

Magnetic resonance imaging (MRI) is diagnostic in more than 95% of cases, but plain films are useful for assessing bone destruction and overall spine alignment [9].

Pyogenic Infection

Fever, back pain, and tenderness constitute the classical triad. Of these, back pain is the most common presenting feature. There can also be extreme stiffness and muscle spasm of the spine and sometimes radicular pain. The white blood cell count is seldom less in 10,000 per milliliter and the erythrocyte sedimentation rate (ESR) not usually less than 20 mm in the first hour (plasma viscosity 1.7). A raised ESR has been found to be the most reliable laboratory test [13]. It is important that diagnostic material be submitted for aerobic, anaerobic, tuberculous, and fungal examination as well as samples being sent for pathological examination in case the cultures prove negative. In the presence of significant pyrexia blood cultures may yield the organism, but needle biopsy of the spine under computed tomography (CT) guidance is becoming more widely used. Because 40% of patients in one series had received antibiotics before biopsy, an organism was only isolated in 40%, but the result of biopsy led to a change in management in more than a third of patients [14]. Molecular biological techniques are increasingly used to determine the precise organism.

The mainstay of treatment for pyogenic infections is antibiotic therapy according to the culture and sensitivity of the bacteriological examination. Inpatient intravenous antibiotic administration should be prescribed until the general condition of the patient and blood inflammatory markers improve to the point when antibiotics can be administered orally and the patient may be mobilized and discharged. Spinal infection can be very painful, and a thoraco-lumbar orthosis may have a potent analgesic effect.

Most pyogenic infections develop spontaneous interbody fusion and so late instability is uncommon. In addition the recurrence rate is less than 5%. Pyogenic infection is not usually accompanied by significant abscess formation but, if it is, and particularly with cord pressure signs, then anterior decompression is required. Laminectomy is of no value.

Tuberculous Infection

Just as the febrile infant with septicemia, pyogenic spinal infection and failure to thrive has become uncommon, so too has the old-fashioned Potts' tuberculous kyphosis in the young become rarer in the developed world.

Notwithstanding this, tuberculous spinal infection remains common, particularly in those who are, or have come, from developing countries. In addition, vaccination for tuberculosis is only being taken up by a minority of families. Tuberculosis worldwide still causes more deaths than all other notifiable infectious diseases combined. Spinal disease accounts for almost 60% of all musculoskeletal tuberculosis, and the L1 vertebral body is the most commonly affected. The T10 vertebral body is the most common level for the development of paralysis [15].

Tuberculous spinal infection tends to have an insidious onset with more significant local deformity so that the gibbus in an untreated individual is diagnostic. Paralysis as a presenting feature is also much more common than with pyogenic infection. Inflammatory markers are generally only modestly raised. Biopsy is essential and, as with pyogenic infection, the diagnosis can be clinched either by bacteriological assessment or by examination of histological specimens which, in tuberculosis, demonstrate granulomata, giant cells, and caseation. It is particularly important from the bacteriological point of view to identify the organism and its sensitivities so that appropriate chemotherapy can be prescribed.

Tuberculous spinal infection is particularly rife in countries where acquired immunodeficiency syndrome (AIDS) is prevalent and lowers the resistance of the host to infection. Moreover, resistant mycobacteria are increasingly emerging, making the prescription of appropriate antibiotics more difficult. The drugs available for treatment of tuberculous spinal infection are listed in Table 2.1. Some centers use a combination of four drugs but many centers will use just two drugs for 9 months (Rifampicin and Isoniazid), others adding Streptomycin for the first 3 months [9].

Unfortunately drug treatment is often unsuccessful and patient/parent compliance may be a major problem. Significant abscess formation, cord compression, and increasing kyphosis are the indications for anterior decompression, debridement, and strut grafting (the Hong Kong procedure described by Hodgson and Stock in 1960) [16]. Over the past three decades or so it has become apparent that the presence of a metal implant in the tuberculous spine carries with it no morbidity and so it is now routine for internal fixation to be used when operating on the tuberculous spine.

Table 2.1 Anti-tuberculous drugs

Rifampicin 10–600 mg/kg/day
Isoniazid 5–300 mg/day
Ethambutol 25 mg/day for 2 months then reduce
Pyrazinamide 25 mg/kg/day (max. 2.5 g/day)
Streptomycin 0.75–1.0 g/day 60–90 days, then 1.0 g 2–3 times/week

(See also Chapter 10 of General Principles of Children's Orthopaedic Disease)

For whatever reason, and unlike many other causes of paralysis such as tumor, Potts' paraplegia is much more amenable to surgical intervention with a much greater potential for neurological recovery.

Juvenile Discitis

This is a very interesting condition which tends to affect young children after infancy. The lumbar spine is nearly always the site of disease and the child complains of severe low back pain with a rigid lumbar hyperlordosis, often laterally deviated into a mild scoliosis. No movement of the lumbar spine is possible. The child is miserable but not systemically unwell. There is usually no pyrexia, the white blood cell count is normal but the erythrocyte sedimentation rate/plasma viscosity (ESR/PV) may be modestly raised. The earliest plain film findings are slight narrowing of the disc space at the relevant level with some blurring

of the adjacent vertebral margins (Fig. 2.4). Technetium bone scanning is strongly positive in the region of the adjacent vertebral bodies. However, this does not appear to be an infectious condition and biopsies invariably fail to grow organisms.

The term "discitis" was first coined by Menelaus [17] to describe this disorder characterized by disc inflammation but no primary bone involvement. The Mayo Clinic group also recognized that this was a non-infective condition and thought it might be an autoimmune reaction [18].

With time, further disc space narrowing occurs, but this seldom goes on to spontaneous fusion. Symptomatic treatment consists of initial bed rest, followed by a thoracolumbar orthosis (in the ambulatory child). Stiffness and pain may take several months to settle, a frustrating period for child, parents, and doctor.

Arthritis

Early-onset ankylosing spondylitis is very uncommon. The disease appears to be pursuing a more benign course quite naturally. In the 1997 classification of the childhood arthritides, two types may affect the spine, enthesitis-related arthritis and psoriatic arthritis [19]. The childhood form of enthesitis-related arthritis is similar clinically to the adult form and is also strongly linked to the HLA B27 antigen (Fig. 2.5). Sacroiliitis is not diagnostic and only a small minority (15%) have spinal symptoms early on. The condition occurs more frequently in boys with a typical age of onset at about 11 years. It is not uncommon for the first symptom to be hindfoot pain and stiffness.

With psoriatic arthritis, the arthritis tends to appear before the psoriasis. Girls are affected more than boys with age of onset generally under 11 years.

Adolescent Disc Syndrome

This describes disc prolapse in the second decade. It is a similar process of disc degeneration to that which occurs in adults

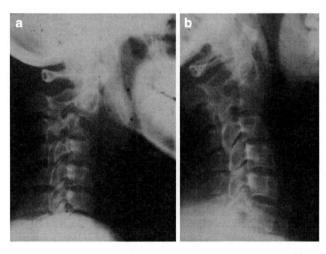

Fig. 2.4 Tuberculosis of the spine. (**a**) Lateral radiograph of the neck of a quadriparetic teenage girl immigrant showing destruction of the third cervical vertebra and a huge retrophalangeal abscess (*arrowheads*) causing spinal cord compression. (**b**) Lateral radiograph of the neck 2 years after anterior debridement, cord decompression, and strut grafting. There was complete resolution of the neurological signs and a solid fusion

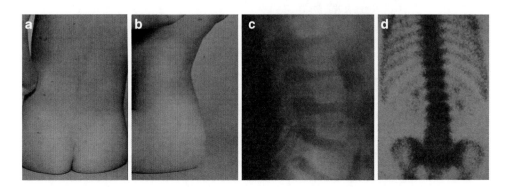

Fig. 2.5 Juvenile discitis. (**a**) Back and (**b**) side views of a 6-year-old boy with a typical rigid hyperlordosis and slight scoliosis produced by muscle spasm. (**c**) Lateral radiograph of the lumbar spine showing L2/3 disc space narrowing. (**d**) Isotope bone scan showing increased uptake in L2 and L3

with dehydration and increasing disc stiffness. There is seldom a discrete herniation, but rather bulging of the nucleus within a contained annulus [20].

In the mid-1990s Battié and his colleagues in Finland looked at the Finnish identical twin cohort, all of whose spines were MRI scanned. There was a remarkably similar distribution of degenerative disease in each of the twins' spines but very importantly, when they were divided into discordant groups as regards physical activity (heavy jobs or contact sports versus a sedentary lifestyle), there was no difference in the severity of degenerative disease between each set of twins [21].

There have been several case reports of children with degenerative disc disease, one involving a girl of 12 whose lumbar spine symptoms were so severe that they warranted an MRI scan which showed multi-level disc degeneration and herniation. Her identical twin sister volunteered for a MRI and it showed similar multi-level disc disease, demonstrating the genetic etiology of the condition [22]. The youngest child we have treated in Leeds was a boy of 4 years.

In the adolescent the predominant symptom is low back pain. Radicular pain and paraesthesia are seldom early symptoms. There is marked lumbar stiffness and very often a sciatic tilt (Fig. 2.6). Otherwise the back pain is mechanical, being worsened by activity and being eased by rest. Forward bending is markedly restricted and often produces a sciatic scoliosis; straight leg raising is also very limited but would appear to be due to hamstring tightness rather than a truly positive straight leg raise test. These clinical features can produce a most unusual gait and it is not at all uncommon for an adolescent to present with all the above features and yet deny severe pain or even have no pain at all. A prolapse in this age group does not produce marked neurological loss in the compromised nerve roots. Sphincter symptoms are very rare. Plain films are normal although spinal posture indicates spasm. The diagnosis is clinched by MRI which shows diffuse bulging of the disc rather than a focal hernia (Fig. 2.7).

Treatment is expectant but recovery is slow and may take 18 months to 2 years. Unless the case is unusually associated with significant neurological dysfunction operative treatment should be withheld. If nerve root decompression is required then the same sort of results can be expected as in the adult. A microsurgical approach should yield an excellent result in 90%.

Sometimes in the adolescent a very large disc prolapse can be seen to resorb as symptoms improve and finally settle.

Spondylolisthesis

Spondylolysis and spondylolisthesis are by far the commonest causes of low back pain in childhood and adolescence [23].

Isthmic Spondylolisthesis

The incidence of spondylolysis (stress fracture in the pars interarticularis) has increased over the past decades as more sophisticated diagnostic radiographic techniques have been used for the child with low back pain. By far the majority of spondylolyses occur at L5 and consequently the slip occurs at the L5/S1 level. Plain films reveal spondylolyses in about 5% of children in the population (Fig. 2.8) with a slippage of about half that rate [24]. If CT scanning with an oblique gantry angle is utilized then the prevalence rate doubles (Fig. 2.9). The defect can also be seen on MRI (Fig. 2.10).

The pain is well localized to the low back, although it may radiate to the buttocks and thighs. Symptoms tend to be worsened by extension of the spine and activity, and reciprocally relieved by rest. There would appear to be a much higher incidence in gymnasts, athletes, ballet dancers, trampolinists, and other flexible athletes, reflecting increased repetitive cyclical movement of the low back during sporting activities [25]. The incidence rises to almost 50% in Eskimos which strongly suggests a genetic factor [26]. Recent research has demonstrated that when lyses occur

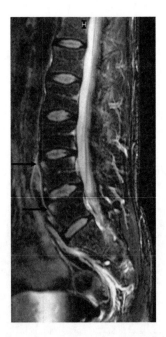

Fig. 2.6 Ankylosing spondylitis. T2-weighted sagittal image of the lumbar spine of a teenage boy showing the oedematous Romanus lesions typical of early disease

Fig. 2.7 Adolescent disc syndrome. (**a**) Back view of a teenage boy with a sciatic scoliosis. Note the erythema ab igne over the left lumbar region due to the application of a hot water bottle for pain relief. (**b**) Axial MRI image of his L5/S1 disc showing a large central disc hernia

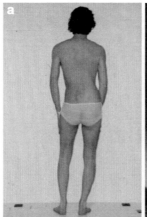
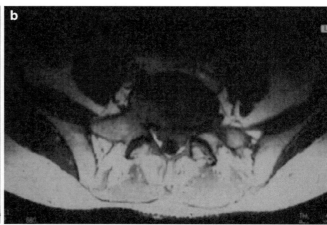

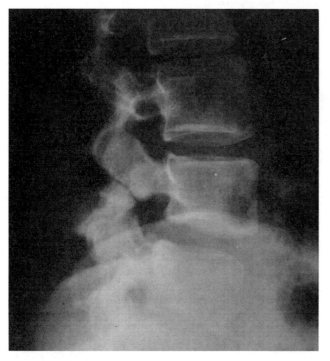

Fig. 2.8 Lateral radiograph of the lumbar spine showing bilateral L4 lyses with a slight L4/5 slip

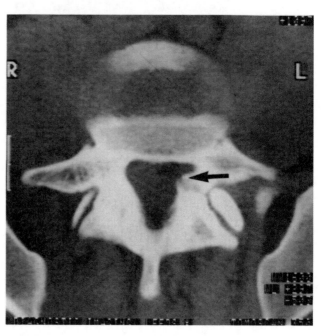

Fig. 2.9 Axial CT scan of L5 showing a lysis on the left side (*arrow*) and sclerosis of the pedicle on the right side, a common combination

either unilaterally or bilaterally the facet joint orientation is significantly more coronal, and this would therefore allow a pincer effect, particularly in spinal extension, thus leading to fatigue failure across the pars [27].

Treatment is expectant and symptoms usually settle with a period of rest from sporting activity or perhaps the intermittent use of a lumbosacral orthosis. Injections of the lytic region under radiographic control using a local anesthetic and a water soluble steroid can also be helpful in more recalcitrant cases. Slippage very seldom exceeds 20–30% and never becomes complete (the isthmic form of spondylolisthesis). Only in the most recalcitrant cases should spinal fusion be necessary.

Dysplastic Spondylolisthesis

This form of spondylolisthesis is more likely to slip progressively, although it is much less common than the isthmic form. The primary problem is hypoplasia or aplasia of the L5/S1 facet joints and so the deformity always occurs at the L5/S1 level. It is not so much a forward slippage but a forward rolling of the L5 vertebra on the top of the sacrum (Fig. 2.11). This can sometimes progress to complete spondyloptosis with L5 sitting on the front of the sacrum and it is in these very progressive slips that prophylactic fusion has a place. Despite the fact that there is no lysis of L5 to leave the back of the spine behind, neurological compromise is rare (see Chapter 4).

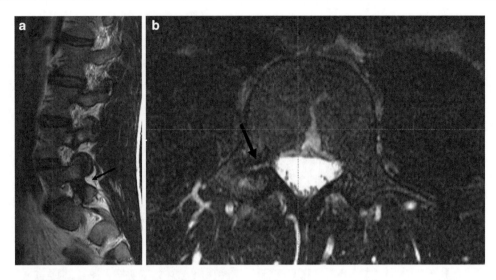

Fig. 2.10 Sagittal and axial MRI views through the fourth lumbar vertebra showing a unilateral lysis (*arrowed*)

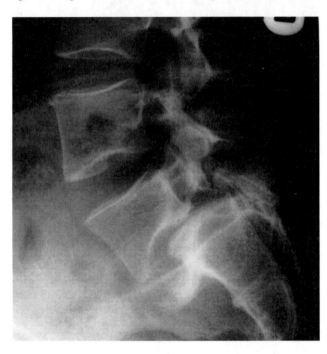

Fig. 2.11 Lateral radiograph of the lumbar spine showing a dysplastic spondylolisthesis with a lordotic-shaped L5 body, reciprocal rounding of the top of the sacrum, and secondary lyses in the back of L5

Tumors

Spinal neoplasms may be grouped into those that occur in bone, in neurological tissue, or in paravertebral tissues.

Intradural Tumors

When spinal cord dysfunction in the child occurs subacutely or chronically, it is most often due to tumor. Tachdjian and Matson [28] have written the most informative article on the subject of intraspinal tumors in children which should be compulsory reading for all orthopaedic surgeons who treat children. They reported on 30 years of experience in Boston. In children the most common intradural neoplasms are gliomas, including astrocytomas and ependymomas. Neuroblastoma is the second commonest neoplasm but the commonest cause of spinal cord compression in the infant. Boys are affected twice as commonly as girls and 50% occur in the first 4 years of life. Slightly more lesions are benign than malignant.

Limp and leg weakness are the chief presenting features; back pain is present in one-third and torticollis in one-fifth. The most important physical findings in order of frequency are pathological reflexes, spastic paralysis, flaccid paralysis, a sensory level loss, a scoliosis in one-third, and muscle spasm. Tachdjian and Matson found an alarmingly high rate of wrong initial diagnosis, these tumors being commonly attributed to poliomyelitis, brachial plexus lesions, muscular dystrophy, and postural torticollis [28]. Fraser et al. [29] found sphincter disturbance in one-fifth. In children under the age of 6, 75% are malignant, falling to 30% over the age of 6.

Back pain tends not to be episodic but characteristically continuous and steadily worsening. Typically, inactivity increases the pain so that patients tend to pace the room at night. Tumors involving the cord tend to have upper motor neurone features and a progressive sensory disturbance, while cauda equina lesions have lower motor neurone features with painless leg wasting. Intramedullary lesions produce a characteristic, suspended disassociated sensory loss with reduction in pain and temperature but normal appreciation of touch; this physical sign is common also in syringomyelia. Vertebral column signs include reduced straight leg raising, decreased lumbar lordosis, and a scoliosis.

Syringomyelia has some similarities with intradural neoplasms and is a chronically progressive degeneration of the spinal cord and medulla, resulting in cavitation and gliosis within the substance of the cord. The condition was first described by Duchenne [30] and there are two pathological varieties: communicating and non-communicating. In the former there is communication between the cavity and the posterior fossa, while in the latter the fluid has another origin, usually from tumor or traumatic paraplegia. Typically, there is sensory dissociation with pain and temperature sensation involved but not touch at the level of the lesion, and weakness and wasting of the muscles of the involved segments. The commonest presenting symptom is pain in the head, neck, trunk, or limbs increased by straining. The cervical spine is the most commonly affected area.

With intradural tumors and syringes plain radiographs may show interpedicular widening and erosion of both neural arches and vertebral bodies locally (Fig. 2.12). Untreated cases can develop intrinsic muscle wasting and clawing of the hands as well as pes cavus. Treatment is by way of posterior fossa decompression (communicating) or cerebrospinal fluid shunting (non-communicating).

Laminectomy with tumor excision and additional radiotherapy for those which are malignant is the treatment of choice and microsurgical techniques are essential, often with a deep and wide laminectomy. It is important that this should be carried out by a neurosurgeon in combination with an orthopaedic spinal surgeon who can then stabilize the spine to prevent the inevitable progressive kyphosis (Fig. 2.2). The prognosis is not appreciably reduced by incomplete excision if radiation treatment is given post-operatively and the 5 year survival for malignant disease is better than 60%.

Tumors of Bone

The common bone-forming tumors in childhood and adolescence are the osteoid osteoma/osteoblastoma and the aneurysmal bone cyst.

Osteoid osteomas and osteoblastomas have the same histological appearance of vascularized osteoid tissue with a central nidus. Osteoid osteomas are cortical or subcortical, surrounded by an area of sclerotic bone, the nidus being about 1 cm in diameter. In contrast, osteoblastomas are medullary and the reactive zone is greater than 2 cm in diameter (Fig. 2.13). They tend to occur in the spine and flat bones. These lesions are painful because of the release of prostaglandins, so symptoms are relieved by prostaglandin inhibitors.

Plain films may appear normal with osteoid osteomas as they are cortical. Radiographs are always abnormal with

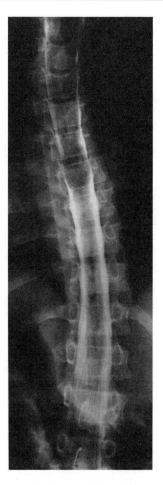

Fig. 2.12 Myelogram of a 12-year-old boy with a mild scoliosis and severe pain, particularly at night. There is marked pedicular widening in the upper thoracic spine going through to the neck and the syrinx extends down into the lumbar region. It proved to be secondary to a malignant glioma

osteoblastoma, particularly enlargement and expansion of the base of the adjacent transverse process. Both lesions are intensely positive on technetium bone scanning.

Delay in diagnosis is common and in one series averaged almost 18 months [31]. The natural history for these lesions is to settle spontaneously but persistence and severe pain merit treatment. Osteoid osteomas can be ablated under radiographic control but the larger osteoblastomas require complete surgical removal.

Aneurysmal bone cysts are of unknown pathogenesis but their large blood-filled spaces are separated by fibrous septa which contain both osteoblasts and osteoclasts. They were thought to be variants of giant cell tumors, but any spinal lesion that looks as though it might be a giant cell tumor is almost always an aneurysmal cyst.

Radiographically they have a "blow-out" appearance with soap-bubble trabeculation (Fig. 2.14), and while their growth may be so rapid as to imply malignancy, they are benign and recurrence is not common. One-fifth of

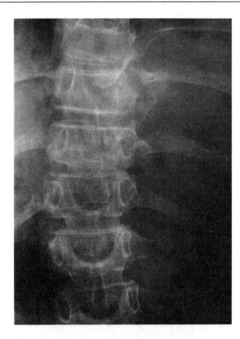

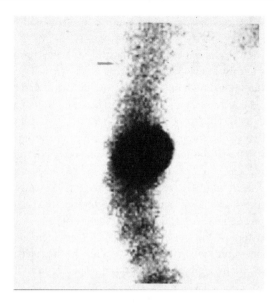

Fig. 2.14 Technetium bone scan showing intense uptake, characteristic of this lesion

Fig. 2.13 Osteoblastoma. Posteroanterior (PA) radiograph of the thoraco-lumbar region in a 14-year-old boy with a mild scoliosis and severe pain at night. The pedicle at T10 on the right side is missing and the lesion extends into the transverse process, the typical site for an osteoblastoma

all aneurysmal cysts are in the vertebral column, most commonly the lumbar region (Fig. 2.15). They tend to occur between the ages of 10 and 15 years [32]. The current

preferred treatment is complete excision of the lesion which may require total vertebrectomy and a strong anterior strut graft.

Eosinophilic granuloma of the spine produces back pain and muscle spasm, tenderness, local spinal rigidity, and often a mild kyphosis. The condition was described first by Calvé [33] in 1925 and in those days the important differential

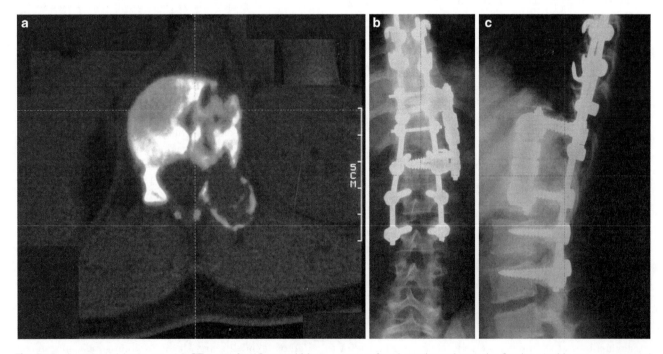

Fig. 2.15 Aneurysmal bone cyst. (**a**) CT scan of a 15 year old boy with severe constant back pain showing the typical blow-out appearance of an aneurysmal bone cyst. (**b**) AP and (**c**) lateral radiographs 2 years after combined anterior and posterior total vertebrectomy with a strut graft and anterior and posterior fixation. At this stage we removed the posterior metalwork; he resumed playing rugby and grew to a height of 6' 6"

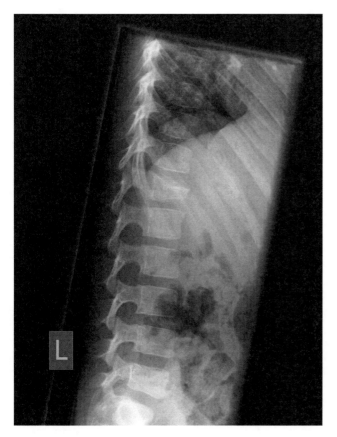

Fig. 2.16 Lateral radiograph showing an eosinophilic granuloma of T12 in the early stages of collapse

diagnosis was Pott's disease. It was not until 1953 that Lichtenstein [34] gave the lesion the name "Histiocytosis X" and integrated eosinophilic granuloma of bone with Letterer–Siwe disease and Hand–Schüller–Christian disease, similar lesions with a common histological pattern [34]. Lesions of the vertebral bodies go through stages of an initial lytic appearance followed by collapse (Fig. 2.16) and then increased sclerosis before recovery to normal height which may take 1–3 years. Radiographically there is a typical vertebra plana appearance of a silver dollar on its edge. Treatment is not indicated but biopsy may be required to distinguish it from osteomyelitis, Ewing's tumor, or malignancy.

References

1. Burgoyne W, Edgar M. The assessment of back pain in children. Curr Paediatr 1998; 8:173–179.
2. Fairbank JCT, Pynsent PB, Poortvleit JAY, Phillips H. Influence of anthropometric factors and joint laxity in the incidence of adolescent back pain. Spine 1984; 9:461–464.
3. Balagué F, Troussier B, Salminen JJ. Non-specific low back pain in children and adolescence: risk factors. Eur Spine J 1999; 8: 429–438.
4. Kewalramani LS, Tori JA. Spinal cord trauma in children; neurological patterns, radiologic features and pathomechanics of injury. Spine 1980; 8:11–18.
5. Bohlmann HH. Acute fractures and dislocations of the cervical spine; analysis of 300 hospitalised patients and review of the literature. J Bone Joint Surg 1979; 61A:1119–1142.
6. Henrys P, Lyne ED, Lifton C, Salciccioli G. Clinical review of cervical spine injuries in children. Clin Orthop 1977; 129:172–176.
7. Cullen JC. Spinal lesions in battered babies. J Bone Joint Surg 1975; 57B:364–366.
8. Dickson RA, Leatherman KD. Spinal injuries in child abuse; case report. J Trauma 1978; 18:811–812.
9. Wilson-Macdonald J. Management of spinal infection. Cur Orthop 2003; 16:462–470.
10. Wedge JH, Oryshak AF, Robertson DE, Kirkaldy-Willis WH. A typical manifestations of spinal infections. Clin Orthop 1977; 123:155–163.
11. Batson OV. The function of the vertebral veins and their role in the spread of metastases. Ann Surg 1940; 112:138–149.
12. Wiley AM, Truator J. The vascular anatomy of the spine and its relationship to pyogenic vertebral osteomyelitis. J Bone Joint Surg 1959; 41B:796–809.
13. Griffin PH, Hooper JC. Vertebral osteomyelitis. J Bone Joint Surg 1976; 58B:258.
14. Rankine JJ, Barron DA, Robinson P, et al. Therapeutic impact of percutaneous spinal biopsy in spinal infection. Postgrad Med J 2004; 80:607–609.
15. O'Brien JP. Kyphosis secondary to infectious disease. Clin Orthop 1977; 128:56–64.
16. Hodgson AR, Stock FE. Anterior spine fusion for the treatment of tuberculosis of the spine. J Bone Joint Surg 1960; 42A: 295–310.
17. Menelaus MB. Discitis—an inflammation affecting the intervertebral discs in children. J Bone Joint Surg 1965; 46B:16–23.
18. Boston HC, Bianco AG, Rhodes KH. Disc space infections in children. Orthop Clin North Am 1975; 6:953–964.
19. Edmonds SE. Juvenile arthritis. In Bulstrode C, Buckwalter J, Carr A, et al., eds. Oxford Textbook of Orthopaedics and Trauma. Oxford and New York: Oxford University Press; 2002:2427.
20. Taylor TK, Akeson WH. Intervertebral disc prolapse: a review of morphologic and biochemic knowledge concerning the nature of the prolapse. Clin Orthop 1971; 76:54–79.
21. Battié MC, Videman T, Gibbons LE, et al. 1995 Volvo award in clinical sciences. Determinants of lumbar disc degeneration. A study relating lifetime exposures and magnetic resonance imaging findings in identical twins. Spine 1995; 20(24): 2601–2612.
22. Obukhov SK, Hankenson L, Manka M, Mawk JR. Case report. Multilevel lumbar disc herniation in 12 year old twins. Childs Nerv Syst 1996; 12:169–171.
23. Dickson RA. Spondylolisthesis. Curr Orthop 1998; 12(4): 273–282.
24. Bailey W. Observations on the etiology and frequency of spondylolisthesis and its pre-cursors. Radiology 1947; 48:107–112.
25. Jackson DW, Wiltse LL, Cirincioner J. Spondylolysis in the female gymnast. Clin Orthop 1976; 117:68–73.
26. Stewart TD. The age incidence of neural arch defects in Alaskan natives, considered from the standpoint of etiology. J Bone Joint Surg 1953; 35A:937–950.
27. Rankine JJ, Dickson RA. An investigation of the facet joint anatomy in spondylolysis. Musculoskeletal Scientific Session 1. Proceedings of the UK Radiology Congress 2008. British Institute of Radiology.
28. Tachdjian MO, Matson DD. Orthopaedic aspects of interspinal tumors in infants and children. J Bone Joint Surg 1965; 47A: 223–248.

29. Fraser RD, Paterson DC, Simpson DA. Orthopaedic aspects of spinal tumors in children. J Bone Joint Surg 1977; 59B:143–151.

30. Duchenne GBA. De l'electrisation localisée, 3rd ed. Paris: JB Bailliere et Fils, Paris; 1872:493.

31. Marsh BW, Bonfiglio M, Brady LP, Enneking WF. Benign osteoblastoma: range of manifestations. J Bone Joint Surg 1975; 57A:1–9.

32. MacCarty CS, Dahlin DC, Doyle JB, et al. Aneurysmal bone cysts of the neural axis. J Neurosurg 1961; 18:671–677.

33. Calvé J. A localized infection of the spine suggesting osteochondritis of the vertebral body, with a clinical aspect of Pott's disease. J Bone Joint Surg 1925; 7A: 41–46.

34. Lichtenstein L. Histiocytosis X; integration of eosinophilic granuloma of bone, Letterer-Siwe disease, and Schüller-Christian disease as related manifestations of a single nosologic entity. AMA Arch Pathol 1953 56: 84–102.

Chapter 3

Spinal Deformities

Robert A. Dickson

Basic Principles

Definitions and Terminology

The spine is normally straight in the frontal (coronal) plane. If it is not, a lateral curvature or scoliosis is present. Scolioses are subdivided into structural and non-structural, according to whether the spine is additionally twisted [1]. Thus structural scoliosis is defined as a lateral curvature with rotation. The important attribute of a structural scoliosis is that it is intrinsic to the spine and may progress with growth to produce a serious deformity that may threaten health and quality of life. By contrast, non-structural curves are secondary to some other factors such as leg length inequality or muscle spasm from a painful focus (e.g., disc prolapse, infection, tumor). Significant progression is seen only occasionally in some curves associated with spinal cord tumor. Other non-structural curves tend to resolve when the underlying problem is dealt with.

In the sagittal plane, it is normal to have lordotic spinal curvatures (curves convex anteriorly) in the cervical and lumbar regions and an intervening kyphosis (a curve convex posteriorly) in the thoracic region. Only if these natural curves are exaggerated or reduced can they become pathological. For instance, the thoracic kyphosis is increased in Scheuermann's disease, otherwise known as idiopathic hyperkyphosis. The lumbar lordosis is characteristically increased in paralytic conditions such as muscular dystrophy or cerebral palsy.

Distinguishing between structural and non-structural scoliosis is not always easy on initial inspection. Most non-structural curves occur lower down in the spine, where the lateral profile is naturally lordotic. If a lateral curvature develops here, for example, secondary to the pelvic tilt produced by leg length inequality, then the presence of a spinal curvature in two planes (lordosis plus lateral curvature) will impose a deformity in the third plane, with resultant spinal rotation (Fig. 3.1). It is for this reason that non-structural lumbar scolioses, secondary to a leg length inequality, are found in large numbers during school screening programs that focus upon minor alterations in spinal shape.

It is conventional to describe scolioses according to their site, direction, and the number of curves present. The site of a curve is determined by the position of its apical vertebra or vertebrae, and thus curves can be, for example, thoracic or lumbar. Curves with apices at T12 or L1 are called thoraco-lumbar and those at C7 or T1 are cervico-thoracic. The direction of curve convexity determines the side of the

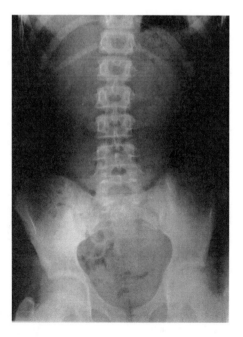

Fig. 3.1 PA view of the lumbar spine and pelvis showing a lumbar scoliosis due to pelvic obliquity secondary to a leg length inequality. There is mild rotation in the upper lumbar region

R.A. Dickson (✉)
Academic Unit of Orthopaedic Surgery, Leeds General Infirmary, Leeds, UK

curve: right thoracic and left lumbar curve patterns are common. Multiple curves are more common than single ones, with the combined right thoracic and left lumbar pattern the most common.

Structural and Non-Structural Scoliosis

When Adams in 1865 [2] described his "forward-bending test," he recognized that the rotational component of the three-dimensional deformity increased with spinal flexion (Fig. 3.2). This remains the favored position for examining patients in scoliosis clinics and in community screening programs. Because the deformity is less evident in the erect position, a mechanical event must take place when the spine flexes to enhance rotation. This provides an important clue to the nature of the underlying deformity of structural scoliosis.

When a postero-anterior (PA) radiograph of a structural scoliosis is examined the lateral curvature is obvious, but the vertebrae within the curve are also rotated, and this direction of rotation is constant: the posterior elements turn into the concavity and the vertebral bodies into the convexity, irrespective of the type or spinal level of the scoliosis. If the spinous processes and the centers of the vertebral

bodies are marked on a PA radiograph, it can be seen that the line joining the spinous processes is shorter than the line joining the vertebral bodies, and thus the back of the spine is shorter than the front (Fig. 3.3). If the back of the spine is shorter than the front in every case of structural scoliosis, then all these deformities are lordotic and there is no such deformity as kyphoscoliosis. This fundamental point was obvious to Adams in the mid-nineteenth century before radiographs were discovered, and his careful cadaver dissections demonstrated the essential lordosis beautifully. The overlong front of the spine readily buckles to the side on flexion, to produce a positive Adams' forward-bending test. It is the three-dimensional nature of this deformity, particularly with reference to the abnormal lateral profile, that holds the key to understanding the clinical features, behavior, and treatment of idiopathic scoliosis.

"Structural" scolioses resulting from solitary congenital hemivertebrae tend to exist in the coronal plane only and exhibit no rotational prominence on forward bending and no rotation on the PA radiograph: the sagittal profile is not affected. Similarly a true lordoscoliosis is produced by leg length inequality, by the combination of coronal and sagittal plane curvatures, but the sagittal profile is not abnormal and progressive buckling does not develop.

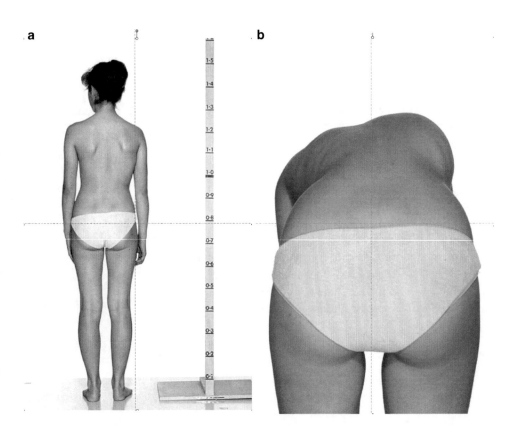

Fig. 3.2 (a) Erect and (b) forward-bending views of a teenage girl with a right thoracic idiopathic scoliosis. The rib hump is much bigger in the forward-bending position

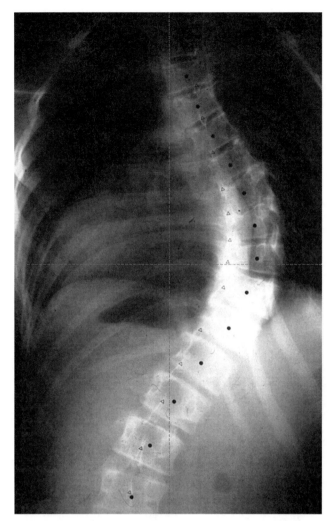

Fig. 3.3 PA radiograph of a right thoracic idiopathic scoliosis. The center of the vertebral bodies has been marked with *solid dots* while the tips of the spinous processes have been marked with *hollow triangles*. It can be seen that a *line* down the back of the spine would be shorter than a *line* down the front confirming the presence of a lordosis

radiograph of a structural scoliosis is examined and the vertebrae that are maximally tilted at the top and bottom of the deformity are selected, lines can be drawn along their upper and lower borders, respectively. These lines subtend an angle referred to as the Cobb angle, and it is a standard practice to measure the deformity of structural scoliosis in this way (Fig. 3.4).

If the deformity is only in two planes, e.g., a solitary hemivertebra, then this angle accurately reflects the shape of the spine. However, the more the spine has twisted the less satisfactory it becomes because the vertebrae within the structural scoliosis are rotated and the PA projection becomes an oblique view of the deformity, with each vertebra being portrayed in a different degree of obliquity (Fig. 3.5). Of course, the direction of rotation of the posterior elements indicates that the deformity is unquestionably lordotic, but it does not say by how much. Meanwhile, the lateral view is another oblique view of the same deformity, this time spuriously suggesting a kyphosis, which is really the scoliosis seen in another plane. In simple terms, therefore, altering the plane of projection changes our perception of a curve's magnitude and shape.

This can be simply verified by inspecting, say, a coat hanger (Fig. 3.6). If the long side (hypotenuse) is vertical, and the hook points due east or west, the angle subtended will be maximal (if we look in a north–south direction), whereas if the hook points north or south the appearance is that of a straight line—i.e., there is no deformity present. As the hook is moved from either due east or west round to north or south,

The Size of the Deformity

Because the deformity exists in three dimensions each vertebra occupies a different position in space relative to its neighbors. *Planes are two-dimensional, and there is therefore no one plane that adequately describes the deformity.* By contrast, if the spine is straight in the coronal plane, a lateral radiograph can be used to measure the amount of cervical or lumbar lordosis and the amount of thoracic kyphosis. Angles are planar measurements and, as no one plane can assess structural scoliosis, the deformity cannot be described by an angular measurement [3]. Cobb [4] was aware of this, but in an effort to assess his patients and their response to treatment he devised the angle that bears his name. If a PA

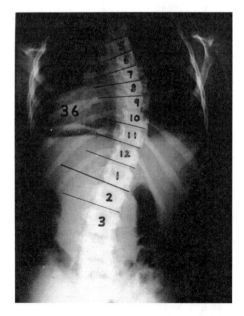

Fig. 3.4 Measuring the Cobb angle. PA radiograph of a right thoracic curve. It can be seen that the sixth thoracic vertebra and the first lumbar vertebra are maximally tilted. These are the end vertebrae. The *lines* along these vertebrae subtend the Cobb angle which in this case is 36°

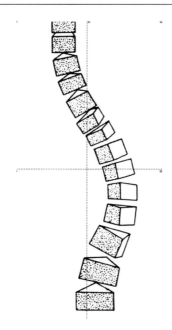

Fig. 3.5 A diagram to show that each vertebra within the structural curve is tilted and rotated and so there is no one plane that can register the entire deformity

the angle subtended steadily decreases. Stagnara was aware of this and devised a radiograph to be taken truly PA to the apical vertebra [5]. If, for example, the apical vertebra was rotated 30° from neutral about a vertical axis, then the radiograph beam was similarly rotated to ensure that this vertebra appeared truly PA. This *plan d'election* is the plane of projection illustrating the largest deformity. A 90° rotated film reveals the true curve apex lateral and unmasks the essential lordosis (Fig. 3.7). Using Stagnara's principle, it is possible only to obtain true PA and lateral projections of one vertebra at a time and excessive radiation would be needed to build up a three-dimensional radiographic picture of a growing child's deformity.

With these limitations, there is much to learn qualitatively if not quantitatively from the PA projection of the patient's spine. In the coronal plane, above and below the structural curve, there are compensatory curves that straighten the spine. These are convex the opposite way to the structural curve and are referred to as "compensatory scolioses." If we consider the direction of rotation of the primary structural scoliosis and its two compensatory curves, it will be seen that for a single curve—e.g., a right thoracic curve—the spinous

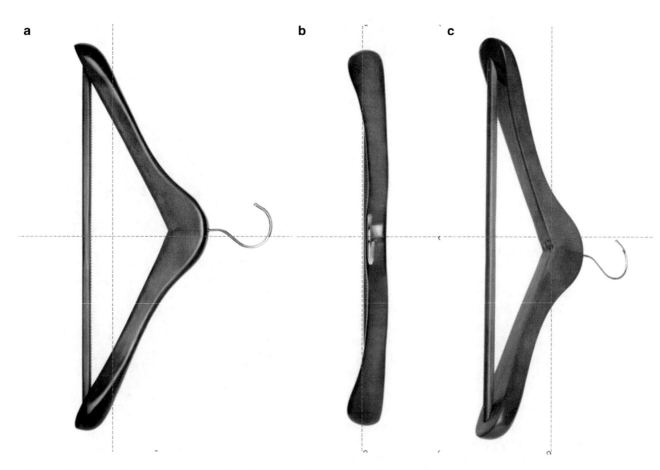

Fig. 3.6 Three views of a coat hanger showing how the angle varies according to the plane of projection

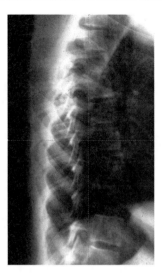

Fig. 3.7 True lateral radiograph of the apical vertebra of a thoracic scoliosis demonstrating the lordosis

processes are rotated toward the left in the region of the structural curve in addition to the first segment or two of the compensatory curves above and below (Fig. 3.4). Bearing in mind that posterior element rotation into the curve concavity implies lordosis, and the reverse kyphosis, the direction of rotation in the compensatory curves is now the opposite of the structural curve—i.e., the compensatory curves are convex left and the posterior elements are also rotated to the left. Thus these so-called compensatory scolioses are kyphoses. This is not surprising because the structural curve is a lordoscoliosis and ought to be balanced in three dimensions above and below by asymmetric kyphoses.

On the PA radiograph of a double-structural right thoracic and left lumbar curve there is no intervening kyphosis between the two structural curves (Fig. 3.8), but there are kyphoses above the upper and below the lower one. Triple- or multiple-curve patterns also exist, and the PA radiograph then shows that the entire spine from top to bottom is lordotic. Thus much about the three-dimensional shape of the spine in structural scoliosis can be inferred from a single PA spinal radiograph.

Classification of Spinal Deformities

The following is a brief classification based upon the recommendations of the Scoliosis Research Society [6]:

1. Idiopathic
2. Congenital
3. Neuromuscular
4. Neurofibromatosis

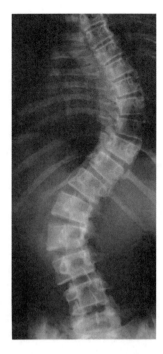

Fig. 3.8 PA radiograph of a right thoracic and left lumbar double-structural scoliosis. The neutral vertebra is T11 and above and below the direction of rotation indicates the presence of lordoses

5. Mesenchymal disorders
6. Trauma
7. Infection
8. Tumors
9. Miscellaneous

Idiopathic spinal deformities are divided into two broad categories: scoliosis and kyphosis. Idiopathic scoliosis is further subdivided into two types according to the patient's age at disease onset—early onset (before the age of 5 years) and late onset (after the age of 5 years). The age distinction is important because it is only with early-onset deformities that health can be jeopardized [7]. Late-onset scoliosis gives cause for concern about appearance rather than health, although there may be social and psychological disadvantages.

Idiopathic kyphosis is Scheuermann's disease, and there are two types according to site. Type I is typically mid-lower thoracic hyperkyphosis, apical about T8–T9, whereas type II Scheuermann's disease is in the thoraco-lumbar or upper lumbar spine and is referred to as "apprentice's spine" as it can be associated with a more vigorous lifestyle.

Congenital spinal deformities are broadly divisible into two groups: bone and spinal cord deformities. Congenital bone deformities are produced by congenital bony anomalies—either failures of formation (hemivertebrae or wedged vertebrae) or failures of segmentation (congenital fusions or bars across disc spaces). When there is a hemivertebra on one side and a unilateral bar on the other, the prognosis is particularly bad because growth leads inexorably to severe progression.

Congenital spinal cord deformities include the spina bifida and myelodysplasia syndromes. The underlying anomaly is present before birth, but the prognosis for deformity depends heavily on the degree of paralysis. Congenital kyphosis in myelomeningocele is always associated with complete paralysis from the waist down, whereas the time of onset and ultimate severity of the more common paralytic-type lordoscoliosis with pelvic obliquity are proportional to the level and severity of paralysis.

These congenital spine deformities are often associated with spinal dysraphism (e.g., diastematomyelia, tethered filum, spino-cutaneous fistula), which may further jeopardize spinal cord function (see Chapter 4 of Children's Neuromuscular Disorders).

Neuromuscular spinal deformities include conditions such as cerebral palsy, poliomyelitis, Friedreich's ataxia, and the muscular dystrophies. The typical paralytic lordoscoliosis with pelvic obliquity occurs in proportion to the severity of the neurological problem.

Neurofibromatosis deformities are either scoliosis or kyphosis and can be of early onset and very progressive.

Mesenchymal disorders refer to those heritable disorders of connective tissue (e.g., brittle bone disease and Marfan's syndrome), mucopolysaccharidoses, skeletal dysplasias, and metabolic bone diseases in which spinal deformities occur.

Traumatic spinal deformities can be produced by trauma to the spine itself (fracture, fracture-dislocation, or secondary paralysis) or can result from extra-spinal trauma such as damage to the chest or abdominal wall from surgery, burns, or retroperitoneal fibrosis.

Infection, which may be pyogenic or tuberculous, typically produces kyphotic deformities.

Deformities associated with tumors may be caused by the tumor itself or by its treatment. Non-structural deformities are produced by associated muscle spasm, whereas idiopathic-type scolioses are produced by intradural tumors, probably by a neuropathological mechanism. The widespread laminectomy used to excise the neoplasm can produce progressive kyphosis in the growing spine.

A number of other conditions, such as congenital anomalies of the upper extremity, juvenile idiopathic arthritis, and congenital heart disease, are also associated with a higher prevalence of spinal deformities.

The Pathogenesis of Structural Spinal Deformities

As with all musculoskeletal deformities, structural scoliosis develops as a consequence of both biological and biomechanical factors [8]. Innumerable scoliosis screening programs have shown (as anatomists centuries ago described) that a degree or two of lateral spinal curvature can hardly be considered abnormal. Epidemiological surveys have demonstrated that 10% of normal teenagers have a scoliosis measuring 5° or more. Forty percent of these are due to leg length inequality, but that still leaves a substantial number (6% of all normal children) with a structural scoliosis somewhere in their spine. However, with increasing curve size the prevalence rate diminishes exponentially: 2% have curves of 10° or more and 0.5% a curve of 20° or more [9]. Clearly, something has to be added to "schooliosis" to make it scoliosis, and not surprisingly this problem exists in the sagittal plane. What is perhaps surprising is that the importance of the lateral profile has been largely ignored, despite the pioneering work of Adams [2] and Somerville [10].

More than 20 years ago in Leeds an epidemiological survey involving 16,000 schoolchildren commenced, paying particular attention to the lateral spinal profile. Every year during this 5-year longitudinal survey, measurements such as standing height and bone age were recorded and PA and lateral low-dose radiographs of the spine were taken. A number of children with straight spines at study outset developed idiopathic scoliosis. Analysis of their initial lateral profiles demonstrated that the lordotic sagittal plane abnormality preceded the lateral spinal curvature, so confirming its crucial etiological significance [11] (Fig. 3.9).

When a true lateral radiograph of the apex of an idiopathic thoracic scoliosis is compared with a lateral view of the apical region of a patient with type I Scheuermann's hyperkyphosis, the deformities in the sagittal plane would appear to be exactly the opposite of idiopathic scoliosis (Fig. 3.10): in Scheuermann's disease the anterior vertebral height is *reduced* in comparison with posterior height and Schmorl node formation is situated anteriorly in the growth plate. Idiopathic scoliosis and Scheuermann's disease have therefore considerable similarities: both develop in otherwise normal, healthy children with a similar community prevalence and familial trend [12].

The thoracic kyphosis varies during late childhood and adolescence: in the prepubertal phase it reduces appreciably, only to be regained a year or two before maturity. It is while the kyphosis is reducing in the prepubertal phase, when girls are at their peak adolescent growth, that they are most prone to develop idiopathic scoliosis. Boys, with their constant growth velocity at this age, are relatively protected. However, when their thoracic kyphosis increases just before maturity boys are at their peak adolescent growth period. This may explain why girls are more prone to scoliosis and boys to Scheuermann's disease. Clinically, idiopathic scoliosis presents during adolescence or even childhood while Scheuermann's disease presents a year or two before maturity.

Fig. 3.9 (**a**) PA radiograph of a mild idiopathic scoliosis which developed 2 years into a prospective epidemiological survey. (**b**) PA radiograph at the start of the study showing a straight spine. (**c**) Lateral radiograph at the start of the study showing the primary lordosis

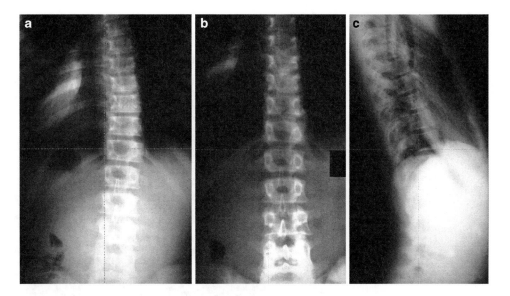

Fig. 3.10 (**a**) True lateral radiograph of the apex of an idiopathic thoracic curve showing vertebral bodies longer at the front than at the back. (**b**) Lateral tomogram of the apex of a Scheuermann's deformity showing reduced height at the front of the vertebrae

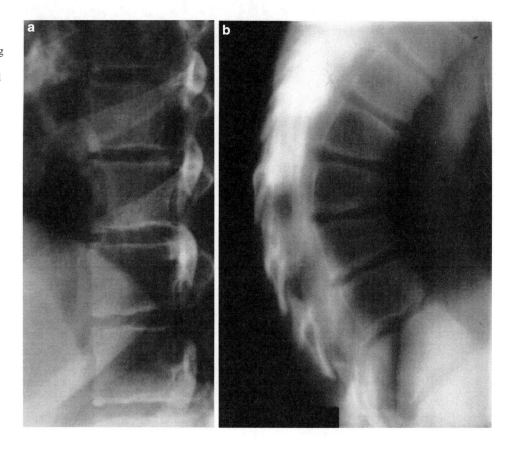

Interestingly, two-thirds of all patients with type I thoracic Scheuermann's disease also have coexistent idiopathic scoliosis, but several segments lower down in the compensatory lumbar hyperlordosis (Fig. 3.11). As the thoracic hyperkyphosis increases, so does the compensatory lumbar hyperlordosis, and the latter readily buckles to the side to produce the scoliosis. Two similar deformities in one adolescent, differing only by their sagittal plane direction, are most unlikely to have different etiologies. The deformities of idiopathic scoliosis and Scheuermann's disease represent the extreme ends of the spectrum of lateral profile, with so-called normal individuals somewhere between.

Fig. 3.11 (**a**) Lateral radiograph of the spine of a patient with thoracic Scheuermann's disease. (**b**) PA radiograph of the same patient showing an idiopathic lumbar scoliosis

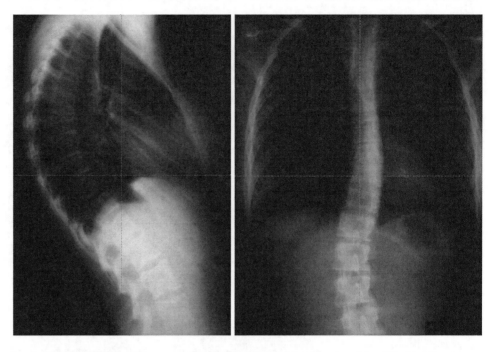

The orientation of the posterior facet joints in the transverse plane allows an axis of spinal column rotation in the sagittal profile of the spine to be constructed (Fig. 3.12). This axis runs behind the cervical and lumbar lordoses, but in front of the thoracic kyphosis. In the transverse plane, vertebral shape is interesting: the cervical and lumbar vertebrae are broad from side to side and short from front to back; the thoracic vertebrae are heart-shaped—much longer from front to back than from side to side and almost pointed anteriorly (Figs. 3.13 and 3.14). Thus the cross-sectional shape of the vertebral column can be considered as triangular or prismatic, with the apex of the prism posterior in the cervical and lumbar regions but anterior in the thoracic region. When a prismatic-shaped structure flexes toward an apex, it buckles much more readily than when it flexes toward a base.

The spine does not stop growing until the middle of the third decade when vertebral endplate growth cartilage can no longer be seen. Therefore, although the spine does not grow appreciably in vertical height after fusion of the long-bone epiphyses, any tendency toward spinal deformity can be accommodated by an alteration of vertebral shape. This accounts for spinal deformities progressing, albeit slowly, after apparent cessation of growth.

Meanwhile, the vulnerable cervical and lumbar lordoses, being in front of the axis of spinal column rotation, have inbuilt protection mechanisms to resist buckling. The bases of the prisms are anterior and the flexibility of the neck and low back allows them to become frankly kyphotic before the limit is reached. They are also protected by the pay-out of powerful paraspinal muscles although, when that fails as in paralytic disorders, a typical collapsing lordoscoliosis is rapidly produced. Finally, the cervical and lumbar lordoses

are top and bottom of the column and buckling tends to occur in the middle, which is precisely where idiopathic thoracic scoliosis and type I Scheuermann's disease occur.

Established engineering laws (Euler's laws) govern column buckling: in this respect, critical load, the modulus of elasticity of the column, the beam length, and the end conditions are all important. For example, both epidemiological and clinical studies have shown that a curve of, say, 40° is more likely to progress than a curve of 20°, all else being equal. This has nothing to do with biology but is purely biomechanical: the more a column has buckled the more likely it is to continue doing so. Similarly, the taller a column the more readily it will buckle, and it is interesting to note that children with idiopathic scoliosis are significantly taller than their straight-backed age- and sex-matched counterparts. There is also evidence that their spines are more slender [13].

The question of critical load is very important. In simple terms, if the spine has any inherent weakness it will buckle more readily, earlier, and more severely. This is recognized in the etiological classification. In conditions such as brittle bone disease or neurofibromatosis, bone is characteristically dystrophic and less strong. In brittle bone disease, bone fractures readily, whereas in Von Recklinghausen's disease bone characteristically grows dystrophically (vertebral scalloping, widened intervertebral foraminae, penciled ribs). The critical load to the spine is therefore increased at bone level and, not surprisingly, in both these disorders there is an earlier onset of spinal deformity and a greater potential for progression. The deformity produced is, however, the same as that occurring in idiopathic cases—i.e., either a lordoscoliosis or a kyphosis.

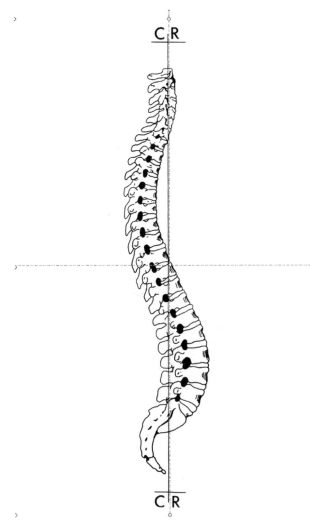

Fig. 3.12 The axis of spinal column rotation (CR) runs in front of the thoracic kyphosis and behind a lumbar lordosis

promotes the development of severe spinal deformities of the idiopathic type. Failure may be at neuromuscular level, i.e., the spinal guy ropes become inadequate, and the weaker they are the more evident is the spinal deformity. In cerebral palsy, the incidence and extent of the paralytic spinal deformity increase with the severity of the neuromuscular deficit.

The spinal column therefore obeys the laws of elementary mechanics but biological factors account for the variability in clinical response [14].

Idiopathic Scoliosis

Idiopathic scoliosis can develop at any time during spinal growth. There are two phases when skeletal growth is particularly rapid—infancy and adolescence—while in the intervening juvenile period growth velocity is relatively constant. Idiopathic scoliosis is thus most prevalent during infancy and adolescence. James in 1954 [15] subdivided idiopathic scoliosis into infantile, juvenile, and adolescent types according to the time of onset but few of his patients belonged to the juvenile-onset group. Long-term follow-up studies of untreated idiopathic scoliosis show considerable disadvantage for those with large deformities not only because of cardiopulmonary morbidity and mortality [16] but also because of social and psychological deprivation [17]. Management of these patients became focused on the concept that curve size must not be allowed to progress excessively with growth: a Cobb angle threshold of 60° became the norm and surgical treatment imperative if this was exceeded.

While the data from these long-term follow-up studies were not flawed, the inferences drawn sometimes were: the size of the deformity attracted attention rather than the age of onset. For example, if one 16-year-old girl has a 50° and another a 100° deformity then, all things being equal, the

Euler's laws allow failure at the soft tissue level also: in Marfan's and Ehlers–Danlos syndromes, ligamentous laxity

Fig. 3.13 The transverse plane geometry of vertebrae resembles prisms. (**a** and **b**) In the cervical and lumbar regions these vertebrae are lordotic in the sagittal plane and prismatic in the transverse plane with the bases of the prisms directed anteriorly, a rotationally stable configuration. (**c**) In the thoracic region the vertebrae are kyphotic in the sagittal plane and prismatic in the transverse plane, this time with the base posteriorly and the apex anteriorly, a very unstable situation rotationally

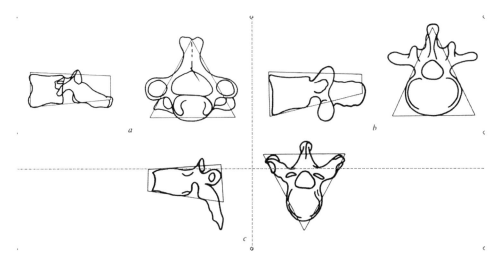

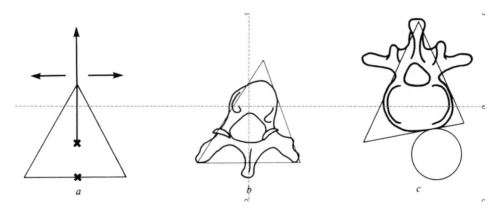

Fig. 3.14 (**a**) If a symmetrical prism was flexed toward its apex it could rotate to either direction. (**b**) The thoracic prisms are not however symmetrical, being constantly grooved on the left side by the pulsations of the descending thoracic aorta such that the apex of the prism is to the right of the median sagittal plane and therefore the prismatic column will tend to rotate to the right. (**c**) In the lumbar region the abdominal aorta is to the left of the median sagittal plane and thus rests against the left side of the base of the lumbar prism. This favors left-sided rotation of the lumbar spine

greater deformity probably started earlier: the age of onset is the crucial issue. The cardiopulmonary implications of scoliosis illustrate this well. At birth the lungs are not simply mini-versions of the adult: rather, they comprise a small number of alveoli which reduplicate until the adult number is achieved by the age of 5 years (Fig. 3.15). Should anything interfere with this process, permanent pulmonary damage can result, leading later to cardiopulmonary dysfunction. A significant thoracic scoliosis with its attendant chest asymmetry may be a critical damaging factor. Branthwaite in 1986 [7] showed that, if the onset of the deformity occurred after the age of 5 years, there was no significant cardiopulmonary compromise no matter how large the Cobb angle. By contrast, the younger the child with scoliosis the greater

is the susceptibility to subsequent heart and lung problems. Clinically, therefore, it is better to consider only two types of idiopathic scoliosis: early onset (before the age of 5 years) and late onset (after the age of 5 years) [1].

Late-Onset Idiopathic Scoliosis (After 5 Years of Age)

This is largely a question of deformity and appearance as there are few health consequences. It is not associated with an increased prevalence or severity of back pain, although when the scoliotic back does become painful, symptoms

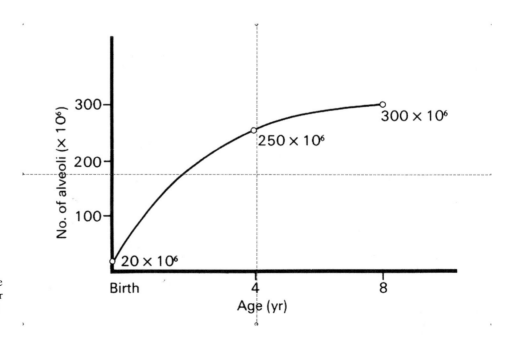

Fig. 3.15 Graph showing the reduplication of the alveolar tree from birth. Almost the full adult complement is reached by the age of 4 but it is the increased number in the first year or two of life that is crucial

are more recalcitrant than with a straight back. The condition, however, should not be regarded simply as cosmetic, as the deformity may have a major impact on the quality of life [17]. It is particularly distressing when an adolescent presents with a deformity so severe that, even with optimal treatment, a significant residual deformity remains for life. Although nowadays fewer such cases attend scoliosis clinics for the first time, curve size at presentation remains a concern and continues to fuel the debate about the value of routine school screening.

When screening was introduced curve size was the dominant consideration. Routine screening has been used for a variety of medical conditions, from which much has been learnt and guidelines and criteria laid down [18]. An important prerequisite is that the natural history of the condition should be adequately understood. Screening for scoliosis has major financial implications and it is pointless to identify thousands of minor cases if progression can neither be anticipated nor prevented. Recent years have shown a progressive loss of confidence in any form of conservative treatment, with many studies struggling to differentiate the effects of treatment from the natural history.

Some countries still insist upon regular routine school screening for scoliosis using some quick measure of rotational asymmetry of the torso on forward bending, such as the scoliometer, but there is a move away from compulsory screening until the natural history is better understood. However, early detection is clearly important, and national orthopaedic associations and scoliosis societies have a responsibility to increase awareness among both lay and medical colleagues of the need for early recognition and prompt referral [9].

An important by-product of school screening programs has been a better understanding of normality and abnormality, of incidence and prevalence rates, curve patterns, and familial trends [19]. Some evidence suggests that the condition is pursuing a more benign course, with lower prevalence and less likelihood to progress [11].

Clinical Features

Patients with late-onset idiopathic scoliosis present with truncal asymmetry and the rotational deformity is usually the most obvious: thoracic deformities present as a rib hump (Fig. 10.8) and thoraco-lumbar or lumbar deformities as a loin hump. Lower curves are associated also with waist asymmetry, an increased flank recession on the concave side, and a flattening of the waist on the convex side. As a result, the hip on the concave side appears unduly prominent and this can be as cosmetically obvious as a rib hump (Fig. 3.16).

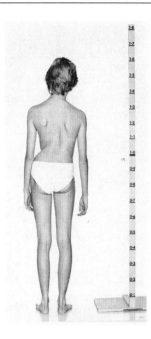

Fig. 3.16 Back view of a teenage girl with an idiopathic lumbar curve showing marked waist asymmetry

Most patients referred to scoliosis clinics are adolescent females. There is a fairly even sex ratio for very small curves detected by screening, but a steep rise in the female/male ratio with increasing curve magnitude. Patients and parents are frequently alarmed by a Cobb angle of 30–40°, and many feel a sense of guilt that they did not recognize the problem earlier. There are two principal reasons for this. First, adolescence is an emotional time and, whereas parents are used to seeing their infants and young children nearly naked, they seldom so see their adolescent children. Although adolescent girls rarely see their own backs, they notice the more prominently developing breast on the side opposite the curve convexity associated with a twisting torso. Second, curve size is more appreciable radiographically: the spinal column has to undergo a certain amount of buckling before this adversely affects the shape of the outer surface of the body. Although this may delay presentation, it has a surgical advantage. If the deformity does not significantly alter surface shape until the Cobb angle reaches 30°, the surgeon does not have to reduce the deformity to much less to make it cosmetically acceptable.

Pain is not a feature of idiopathic scoliosis, although some fatigue discomfort over the rotational prominence may occur. Any suspicion of more significant pain demands further investigation, particularly if there is any suggestion of night pain when neoplasm or a syrinx must be excluded (see Chapter 2). The use of magnetic resonance imaging (MRI) in progressive idiopathic deformities has shown a syrinx to be much more common than previously thought (Fig. 10.12). The usual curve patterns of single right thoracic, single left thoraco-lumbar or lumbar, or double right thoracic and left

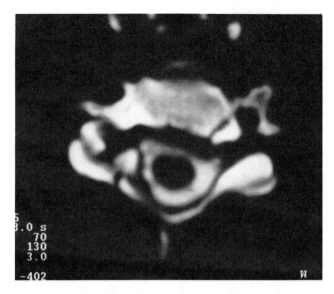

Fig. 3.17 Axial MRI scan through the cervical spine showing a large syrinx in the spinal cord

In idiopathic scoliosis, the neurological examination should be normal. In congenital scoliosis there may be additional spinal dysraphism and the overlying skin in the midline may be the site of a dimple, sinus, nevus, hemangioma, or hairy patch. Furthermore, spinal dysraphism may cause a short so that wasted leg on one side so that a full neurological assessment is essential.

At the conclusion of the history and physical examination, it is useful to obtain a permanent record of surface shape (Fig. 3.18). The deformity buckles further on forward bending and patients should be assessed in flexion as well as upright.

Radiographic Assessment

Too many radiographs are taken of patients with idiopathic scoliosis. At presentation, the patient should have one full set of spinal films, including antero-posterior (AP) and lateral views of the spine from C1 to S1 inclusive. Their principal purpose is to exclude a congenital spine deformity or other relevant feature. As patients present with problems of surface shape, the only certain way of excluding a congenital scoliosis is radiographic. Patients with an intradural tumor or syrinx may appear to have an idiopathic deformity and only radiographs of the whole spine will reveal widening of the interpedicular distance or flattening of the internal pedicular surface. Syrinxes tend to be cervical, reinforcing the need to view the cervical spine. Although emphasis is placed upon isotope scanning for painful scoliosis to exclude

thoraco-lumbar/lumbar (Fig. 3.8) are those we generally see, and any unusual curve pattern, such as a progressive left thoracic curve in a teenager, should arouse suspicion of a possible underlying lesion. If there is any doubt about etiology an MRI must be performed. This is particularly important if surgery is considered because altering spinal shape in the presence of an intradural tumor or syrinx is a recipe for neurological disaster, with a very high rate of paraplegia.

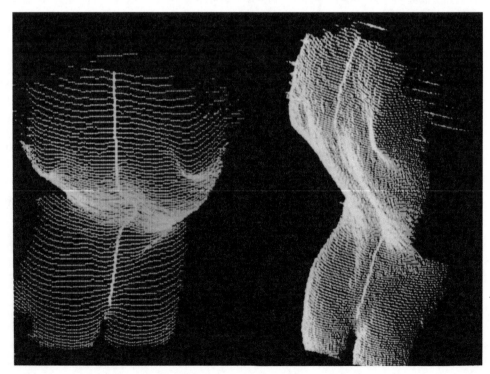

Fig. 3.18 Three-dimensional surface shape measurements recording torso asymmetry in a thoracic scoliosis

osteoid osteoma or benign osteoblastoma, these lesions are usually visible on plain radiographs as an expansion of bone, often with a central lucency, at the junction of pedicle and transverse process on the concave side of the curve apex. A PA view of the left hand and wrist should be obtained in the immature patient to assess bone age.

Measuring the deformity by radiography is controversial, although most scoliosis surgeons continue to use the Cobb angle [4] (Fig. 3.4). Perhaps the most useful single measure on an AP radiograph is the amount of apical rotation at the curve apex. This is a much more accurate index of the patient's chief problem (the rotational component of the deformity). Perdriolle in 1979 [20] introduced his technique using a transparent template over the apical vertebra, with particular reference to the pedicle on the concave side, which is sited more and more toward the concave side, with more and more apical rotation. The amount of rotation is read off in degrees from the template. This measurement of rotation can then be repeated with clinical progression or after surgical intervention. Any differences accurately reflect real change better than the Cobb angle [3]. Unless obscured by metalwork, the convex pedicle is still easily seen after a spinal fusion as it was before.

Radiograph dosage should be kept to a minimum and low-dose techniques are readily available. Good-quality normal-dose radiographs are required at presentation for diagnostic purposes but subsequent radiographs need only be of low dose. Wherever possible, measurement of surface shape should be used in place of radiographs (Fig. 3.18). Although sophisticated techniques are available, they still cannot offer a single overall figure for the patient's deformity.

Treatment

Late-onset idiopathic scoliosis is principally a question of deformity and appearance. What is acceptable depends much more upon the patient and family than the surgeon. Patients' perceptions change during adolescence and "acceptability" may also change with time. This means that, if the deformity were not to change in future, at that moment the patient and family would be happy with the situation. Wise counsel from the scoliosis surgeon is crucial to this decision. Although the surgeon cannot and should not state whether the patient's deformity is acceptable, the advice and information given is essential in helping the family reach a decision [21].

The only way in which spinal shape can be appreciably improved is by major spinal surgery, which may require both anterior and posterior stages. Despite improvements in anesthesia, high dependency care, spinal cord monitoring, and the routine "wake-up" test, there are still definite risks of damaging the spinal cord. Thus acceptability is a balance of risks and rewards; the rewards are a much-improved

spinal shape but the risks include catastrophic neurological deficit. "Acceptability" therefore varies very considerably from deformity to deformity and from family to family as the balance of risk and reward is interpreted differently. A 40° Cobb angle deformity may be so distressing for one patient and family that they would accept significant risks to have it improved, whereas a 70° deformity might be acceptable to another whose concern about one or two major operations and possible paralysis overrides any thought of cosmetic improvement. Although our knowledge of natural history is incomplete, it should be explained that bigger deformities tend to progress more than smaller ones, and more immature patients have a greater progression potential than those approaching maturity. As the spine does not stop growing until the middle of the third decade, it is unwise to consider that progression potential is exhausted when the bones of the hand and wrist reach maturity. Under the responsible guidance of the surgeon and with repeat consultations, often over many years, it is usually possible for the patient, family, and surgeon to reach the correct joint therapeutic decision.

Once acceptability has been decided upon, the management of late-onset idiopathic scoliosis is relatively straightforward. If the deformity is acceptable, then the objective is to preserve this acceptability through the remainder of growth by conservative management. If the deformity is unacceptable, the objective is to restore acceptability and maintain it through the rest of growth by operation.

Conservative Treatment

From the time of Hippocrates various orthotic devices have been worn in the belief that progression of an idiopathic scoliotic deformity could be slowed or prevented. The first popular orthosis was the Milwaukee brace, a cervico-thoraco-lumbar-sacral orthosis introduced by Blount [22] for the postoperative management of poliomyelitic curves. The Milwaukee brace was believed to work by three-point fixation—above, below, and over the apex of the deformity. There was a pelvic mold below, with vertical metal uprights going initially to a ring, which exerted upward pressure on the mandible in front and the occipital condyles behind. Problems with dentition and malocclusion led to the use of a simple cervical choker in later models. Slung between the uprights was a pad held just below the apex of the curve posteriorly to complete the three-point fixation. An important feature was that, for thoracic curves, the lumbar lordosis should be obliterated in the brace and consequently some "correction" could be seen when radiographs were taken without and then with the brace on.

However, the brace did not address the three-dimensional nature of the deformity. Nevertheless, it rapidly became the accepted method of treatment and, in its heyday, it would have been almost heretical to suggest a controlled trial of its efficacy. It was also empirical for the brace to be worn for 23 h a day, from diagnosis until after the vertebral ring apophyses had fused. As spinal growth continues, albeit very slowly, after limb growth, has ceased for a sustained effect to be achieved, the brace would have to be worn until the age of 25 years [23]! Furthermore, it was assumed that children wore their braces assiduously until Houghton et al. [24] showed, by using compliance meters, that they only wore them for a small fraction of the prescribed time: a major disappointment for brace protagonists!

Thresholds for treating idiopathic scoliosis evolved: those with a Cobb angle under 20° were observed; those with an angle 30–50° were braced; those with an angle of greater than 50–60° degrees were operated upon. That brace wearing did not modify natural history was not challenged until recently, when a retrospective study showed that no significant benefit was conferred on brace wearers [25]. The same "corrective effect" had been previously achieved with plaster casts, and flattening of the lumbar lordosis in the cast was considered a very important point. When the need for superstructure was challenged and the Boston underarm thoraco-lumbar-sacral orthosis was introduced, the point of flattening the lumbar lordosis to induce thoracic hyperextension was reinforced, as there was now only two-point fixation rather than the previous three-point fixation [26]. There is, however, no doubt that temporary "correction" by brace wearing can be achieved by flattening the lumbar lordosis.

Electro-stimulation of the convex paraspinal muscles was introduced in the 1970s in an attempt to treat idiopathic scoliosis conservatively. Rather like orthotic treatment, it principally addressed the coronal plane and, not surprisingly, no evidence proved its effectiveness.

A prospective randomized controlled trial was needed to determine whether bracing altered the natural history of late-onset idiopathic scoliosis. Unfortunately, a number of logistical reasons prevented this: bracing proponents would not stop bracing and those who had abandoned bracing would not resume it. Randomization was therefore impossible but centers in America and Europe made their cases available so that at least a prospective comparison could be made between bracing, electrical spinal stimulation, and untreated controls [27]. If a Cobb angle increase of 6° was considered a "failure," then failure occurred in 36% of those braced, 52% of the observed group, and 63% of those electrically stimulated. These differences were statistically significant.

However, in the subsequent paper from this study predicting curve progression [28] there was clear evidence that thoracic curves had a much worse prognosis than thoracolumbar or lumbar curves. In reviewing the original brace trial paper [27] we found that the more benign thoracolumbar curves were much more prevalent in the braced group (32%) but occurred in only 19% of those observed,

seriously undermining the trial's validity. A further in-depth review of bracing for idiopathic scoliosis was carried out [29] which revealed no significant benefit from bracing, questioning again whether the natural history of the deformity could be influenced non-operatively in any way. In simple terms if a thoracic hyperkyphosis needs extension (for which extension bracing is very effective), then a lordoscoliosis needs flexion which as we have seen makes the deformity buckle further (Fig. 3.2).

At present patients with acceptable curves are reviewed regularly; if their curves become unacceptable the only effective treatment is surgical. The majority of curves under 30° will either remain the same or improve somewhat; only about one-third progress to unacceptability. Clinical and epidemiological experience suggests that the proportion which proves unacceptable is smaller than 20 years ago and that the condition is becoming more benign. What is required is a careful contemporaneous longitudinal study of natural history to allow us to identify early the group of patients whose curve will progress; early operation could then be tailored. Similarly, the parents of a young child with a benign 20° curve could be reassured that there was little or no risk of progression. Despite much epidemiological work, we are still far from this ideal.

Surgical Treatment

For almost half a century after Hibbs introduced spinal fusion for scoliosis in 1911 [30] correction was achieved by using pre- and postoperative localizer or turn-buckle casts. In the early 1950s Harrington [31] developed the instrumentation that bears his name and operative management gained considerable momentum. Plaster treatment was not required before operation, although casts or braces were prescribed postoperatively for a period of about 6 months. It would be tempting to think that inserting metalwork would enhance correction. However, when Moe in 1958 [14] compared the results of Harrington instrumentation with localizer cast correction, he found no evidence in favor of the instrumentation. Perhaps this is not surprising, as both localizer casting and Harrington instrumentation seek to correct principally by distraction.

In favor of instrumentation, Moe found a much lower rate of pseudarthrosis and a reduction in the duration of cast treatment and bed rest. The pseudarthrosis rate was so high in the early development of spinal fusion surgery that the American Orthopaedic Association demanded an audit review [32], which confirmed the very high rates of pseudarthrosis and loss of correction in 425 cases. Proper selection of the fusion area, the addition of bone graft [4], and facet fusion [30] reduced the pseudarthrosis rate from just over 50% to a much more acceptable 7%.

The strategy of Harrington's instrumentation was to insert on the concave side of the curve a longitudinal distraction rod that was attached to the spine by hollow hooks. The upper hook was inserted under the facet and the lower hook under the lamina. The upper part of the rod was fashioned into a series of consecutive ratchets that would catch on the margin of the hole in the upper hook so that distraction effected a lengthening of the scoliosis (Fig. 3.19). At the same time,

Harrington insisted upon the insertion of a compression system on the convex side, whereby smaller hooks sliding on a threaded rod compressed above and below the curve apex, thus seeking to shorten the convex side while lengthening the concavity.

By alternate distraction and compression, the deformity was corrected and in addition made rigid, thus favoring fusion and reducing the pseudarthrosis rate. Because an

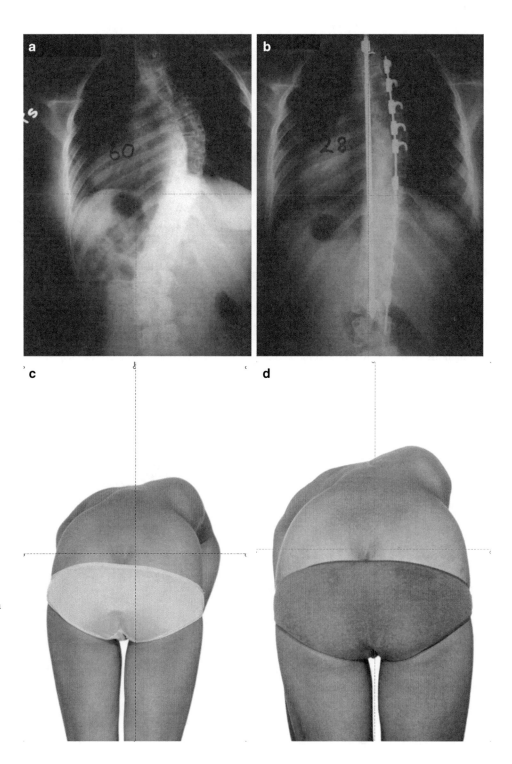

Fig. 3.19 Harrington instrumentation. (**a**) PA view of a thoracic curve measuring 60°. (**b**) Two years after Harrington instrumentation showing a solid fusion and a good correction in the frontal plane. (**c**) Forward-bending view before surgery. (**d**) Forward-bending view 2 years after surgery showing no correction at all in the transverse plane

important part of the deformity was rotational, it was necessary to insert the upper and lower distraction hooks into neutral, non-rotated vertebrae above and below the curve. If the hooks were inserted into the maximally tilted upper and lower end vertebrae then segments of the deformity would be omitted above and, more commonly, below the instrumentation: subsequent growth could lead to buckling beyond the limits of the fusion, so-called adding on. In young children, it was wise to instrument from parallel vertebra to parallel vertebra, thus encompassing not only the scoliosis itself but also the compensatory curves above and below. Combined with meticulous decortication out to the tips of the transverse processes, facet joint excision, and the application of copious autogenous iliac crest bone grafts to induce a massive fusion, this technique became the gold standard of operative scoliosis management, although many surgeons relegated the compression system to an optional extra.

Double curve patterns, e.g., right thoracic and left lumbar, or double thoracic major curves, were dealt with by extending the distraction rod from above the upper curve to below the lower curve, crossing the spine in dollar-sign fashion.

Based upon their considerable experience of Harrington instrumentation, the Minneapolis group devised the King classification of curve patterns to better define the lower end of the fusion, to maintain balance, and to mitigate against adding on [32]. This defines five curve patterns—types 1 and 2 double thoracic and lumbar curves; types 3 and 4 thoracic curves; type 5 double thoracic curve. If a vertical line is drawn upward from the center of the sacrum on an AP view then the lowest vertebra instrumented and fused should be that bisected by this line. They pointed out that the lowest vertebra which needed inclusion in the fusion was often below the lowest neutral vertebra.

However, this King classification is based upon the older Harrington instrumentation and the notion that the postoperative curve size cannot better that measured on preoperative lateral-bending films. Considerably greater correction can now be achieved with modern instrumentation. Furthermore neither the lateral profile nor rotation is taken into account and the classification applies only to adolescent idiopathic scoliosis.

Lenke et al. [33] devised another classification placing greater emphasis on the sagittal plane deformity. This classification has six curve types—(1) single thoracic, (2) double thoracic, (3) double major (thoracic and lumbar), (4) triple major, (5) and (6) thoraco-lumbar and lumbar. This primary classification is modified by the presence and severity of any lumbar curve (based upon the relationship of the lumbar spine to the central sacral line). An additional sagittal thoracic modifier depends upon the lateral profile (the Cobb angle measured on a lateral radiograph). This of course reflects the size of the scoliosis in another plane: the bigger this lateral angle, the bigger the Cobb angle in the frontal plane. However, the Lenke classification is reproducible, appears reliable, and is in wide current use.

In 1982 Luque [34] in Mexico reintroduced the concept of supplementing rods with wires. This technique developed and was practiced extensively early in the twentieth century in Portugal. Sublaminar wires were added to a Harrington distraction rod before Luque realized that the longitudinal rods did not need to be hooked into the spine and developed his twin L-rod system wired at each level on both sides of the spine. His first cases were patients with early paralytic deformities (Fig. 3.20), but the system was subsequently used for idiopathic scoliosis. The addition of sublaminar wires meant that postoperative external support was unnecessary and introduced the concept of segmental correction.

Harrington's instrumentation was a key advance in spinal surgery but it principally addressed the lateral curvature of the spine. Although the patient complained of a rib hump, it was the lateral spinal curvature seen on the radiograph that attracted most attention to the exclusion of the deformity in the other two planes. There were two fundamental problems with this distraction and posterior fusion approach: first, it did not significantly improve the transverse plane deformity and second, in a deformity where the back of the spine is shorter than the front, posterior fusion does not seem logical.

However, as most patients were not far from maturity, they were not penalized by having the shorter side of their spines converted to solid bone, particularly as vertebral bodies are half their adult size at 2 years and virtually full size by 10 years. Most teenagers after Harrington instrumentation and fusion showed an improved Cobb angle, little

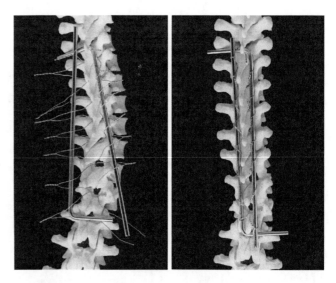

Fig. 3.20 The Luque twin L-rod system. (**a**) The rods are loosely attached with sublaminar wires at each level. The convex L-rod is then cantilevered down to correct the curve. (**b**) A straight spine after final wire tightening

change in their rotational prominence (Fig. 3.19), and little subsequent deterioration.

The situation was very different in the less mature patients: Harrington instrumentation provided only a temporary correction of the Cobb angle, and the posterior tethering fusion of the immature spine led to subsequent buckling with further growth [35]. Adding segmental sublaminar wires to a straight longitudinal rod may not be as advantageous as was initially believed: while providing more rigidity, the sideways pull of the wires behind the axis of spinal column rotation may make rotation worse even though the Cobb angle improves.

Throughout the last two decades further attempts have been made to understand and to rationalize the three-dimensional deformity of idiopathic scoliosis. It was appreciated that there were two essential prerequisites of a surgical procedure: to de-rotate the spine (rather than simply improve the Cobb angle) and to recreate the thoracic kyphosis (to minimize the likelihood of further buckling).

After much experimental work, Dubousset, Cotrel, et al. [36] introduced their intriguing concept of applying a scoliotic rod to the coronal plane of the patient and then turning it through 90° to recreate thoracic kyphosis, while at the same time de-rotating the spine. A second rod on the curve convexity, plus two transverse cross-link metal connections above and below, added considerable stability (Fig. 3.21). In the Cotrel–Dubousset system, the longitudinal rods have a rough outer surface and multiple hooks are used, rather than the simple upper and lower hook of the Harrington assembly. The upper and lower hooks are closed, so that the rod is fitted through a hole in the hook while the intermediate hooks are open, thus allowing easier communication between rod and hook. The multiple hooks allow compression and distraction at different points along the same longitudinal rod. The bulky system reduces the surface bone area available for fusion and is only used to secure the spine temporarily until the associated fusion consolidates. The rigidity of the fixation avoids the need for any postoperative spinal support.

A similar approach was developed in Leeds: if a simple longitudinal Harrington rod with a square-ended lower hook was bent into about 20° kyphosis, then concave sublaminar wires at each level would pull the spine backward, rather than simply sideways. This should permit spinal de-rotation as the thoracic kyphosis is recreated. A pilot study in 50 patients over a 2-year period tested this hypothesis. The initial correction of apical rotation was of the order of 50% and this was sustained at 2 years with no loss of correction [37]. Further experience in 200 cases confirms these excellent results.

It is important to note that the Harrington rod is not distracted after prebending and wire tightening. If the rod were distracted, the deformity would be under tension and the wires could not easily approximate the vertebrae to the rod. Furthermore, injudicious tension could be applied to the contents of the spinal canal. The technique therefore segmentally de-rotates and shortens the spine (Fig. 3.22).

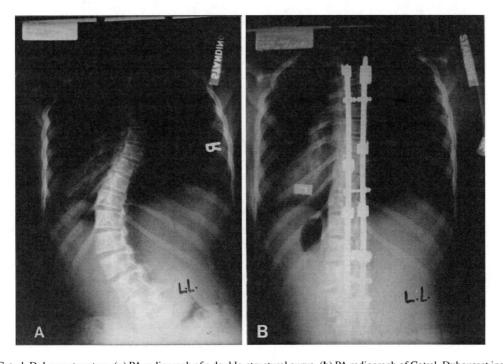

Fig. 3.21 The Cotrel–Dubousset system. (**a**) PA radiograph of a double-structural curve. (**b**) PA radiograph of Cotrel–Dubousset instrumentation

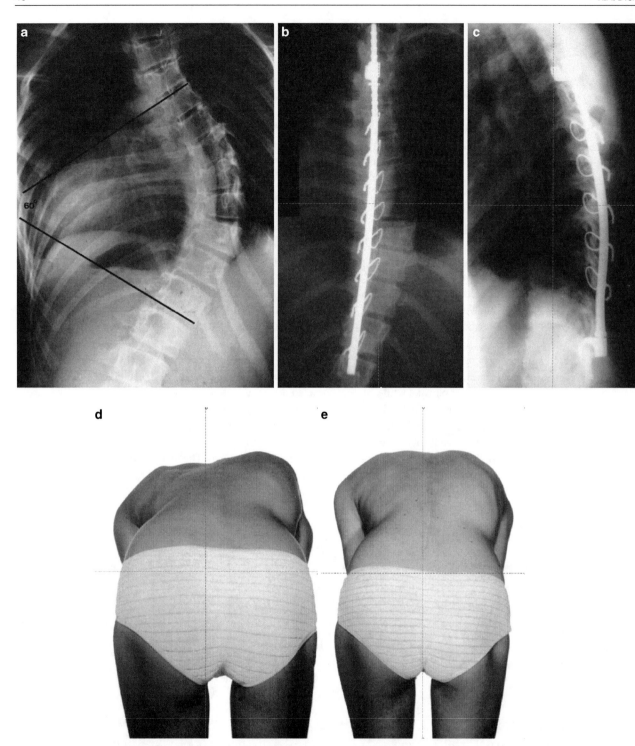

Fig. 3.22 (a) PA radiograph of a 60° right thoracic idiopathic scoliosis. (b) PA radiograph after the Leeds procedure showing a good correction particularly of rib asymmetry. (c) Lateral radiograph postoperatively showing that the sublaminar wires have pulled the concavity back to a kyphotic rod thereby de-rotating the spine. (d) Forward-bending view before surgery showing a sizeable rib hump. (e) Forward-bending view 2 years after surgery showing an excellent and sustained correction of the reason the patient presented in the first place

These original techniques have since been superseded by third-generation instrumentation systems such as the AO Universal spine system and the Moss-Miami spine system and with rods being connected to the spine using mainly transpedicular screws, usually in the lower half of the spine downward, but also sometimes involving the upper thoracic spine (Fig. 3.23).

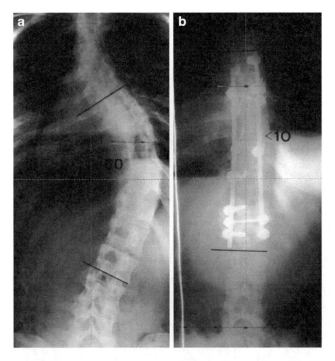

Fig. 3.23 Modern generation posterior instrumentation. (**a**) PA radiograph of a right thoracic curve measuring 60°. (**b**) Postoperative radiograph showing a virtually straight spine

Currently in the United States all idiopathic scolioses at any site and of any severity are dealt with by transpedicular fixation bilaterally from end vertebra to end vertebra. Correction of Cobb angle with these powerful systems is impressive and while some address segmental apical derotation, there is little emphasis on kyphosis restoration to protect the spine from subsequent buckling.

Not only can thoraco-lumbar and lumbar curves be corrected anteriorly but so can thoracic deformities through a thoracotomy, mini-thoracotomy, or indeed thoracoscopically. Anterior fusion is achieved by removing the intervertebral discs at each level to promote interbody fusion: it is important to remove the whole intervertebral disc right back to the posterior longitudinal ligament, not generally possible by mini-thoracotomy or thoracoscopic techniques.

If there is still a residual rib hump at the end of this procedure, it can be further improved by dividing the apical five or six ribs on the curve convexity, just beyond the transverse process. By tucking the lateral cut end under the medial, considerable further cosmetic improvement occurs; this can easily be performed extrapleurally, although a routine pleural drain for 24 h is a good safety measure.

For curves lower in the spine or for double-structural thoracic and thoraco-lumbar/lumbar curves, careful thought is required to decide whether surgery is necessary and which technique is best. Straight posterior metalwork in the lumbar spine may produce an ugly flat-back deformity with a

tendency for patients to lean forward and develop considerable pain. Fusion down to the fifth lumbar vertebra leads to stress concentration on the L5–S1 motion segment and the likelihood of premature degenerative disease at this level. Lordotic contouring of longitudinal metalwork does avoid the flat-back deformity, but a long instrumentation and fusion are still required. Anterior instrumentation and fusion in the low back can avoid flat-back deformity and spare motion segments.

In 1969, Dwyer et al. [38] devised an anterior segmental instrumentation system of transverse vertebral body screws with hollow heads that could receive a braided cable down the curve convexity. When the intervertebral discs and endplates were excised, the convex screw heads could be approximated and then crimped over the cable, thus shortening the long antero-convex side of the deformity. As a result, considerable correction in all three planes was achieved. This system became popular for collapsing paralytic lordoscolioses, but it was not easily accepted for idiopathic thoraco-lumbar or lumbar curves, even though these were the deformities for which the apparatus was devised (Fig. 3.24).

More recently, Zielke's group in Germany markedly improved both the quality of the implants and the instruments used to insert them. His segmental instrumentation and fusion technique is currently favored for thoraco-lumbar or lumbar idiopathic curves [39]. The entire spine may be balanced by applying four apical Zielke screws, so facilitating short fusions. The system utilizes screw heads which are conjoined to a threaded rod; antero-convex shortening is achieved by nut chasing.

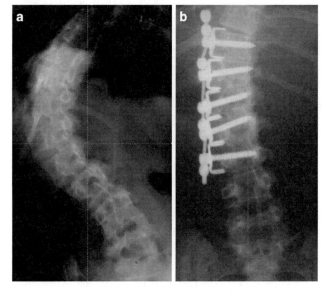

Fig. 3.24 (**a**) PA radiograph of a 90° idiopathic thoraco-lumbar curve. (**b**) PA radiograph showing an excellent correction after anterior Dwyer instrumentation

Fig. 3.25 (**a**) PA radiograph showing a right lower idiopathic thoracic scoliosis with spinal imbalance. (**b**) Postoperative PA radiograph showing an excellent correction of both the curve size and the spinal imbalance

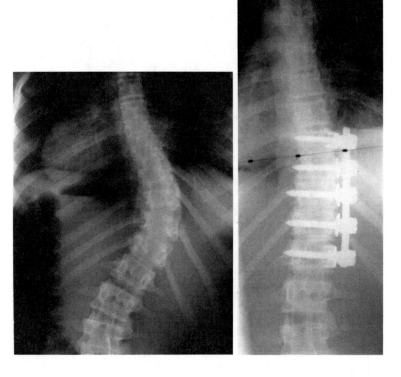

Modern universal spine systems which utilize both anterior and posterior surgical approaches allow excellent correction but are very expensive (Fig. 3.25).

For double thoracic and thoraco-lumbar/lumbar curves, different problems need different solutions. Often either the upper or lower deformity predominates, in which case it should be dealt with as if it were the sole deformity. If the two curves are of similar severity there is merit in dealing only with the lower curve anteriorly, as the upper curve usually improves reciprocally if there is appreciable growth remaining. When the patient is at or near maturity, anterior instrumentation of the lower curve alone may not effect adequate correction of the upper curve (although preoperative traction or side-bending films indicate flexibility). In the mature patient, therefore, it may be best practice to fuse the lower curve anteriorly and the upper curve posteriorly.

As with all other orthopaedic implant procedures prophylactic antibiotics should be used. The risk of neurological injury when correcting major spinal deformity makes it essential to monitor the spinal cord electrophysiologically during the operation, in addition to carrying out routinely a "wake-up test" immediately after tightening or tensioning the instrumentation.

Postoperatively, patients can be mobilized when their wounds are stable. They are usually discharged from hospital within 2 weeks, but it is wise to insist upon 1 month's convalescence at home. Children should be able to return to school 6 weeks after operation, but physical exercise and games should be avoided for 6 months. Swimming and noncontact are then allowed but full mechanical stability should not be assumed before 12 months.

The concept of curve flexibility/rigidity is crucial in scoliosis surgery. For flexible curves up to 60°, a single instrumented posterior fusion usually gives a satisfactory result. Once a curve exceeds 60°, flexibility reduces and, as correction becomes progressively less satisfactory, the risk of inducing tension neurological problems increases appreciably. Understanding the geometry of curve progression helps this fundamental point to be understood. As the primary lordosis buckles out of the sagittal plane, it is progressively more accommodated in the coronal plane, and thus both the lordosis and the true secondary scoliotic deformity increase. Each vertebra in the region of the curve apex becomes progressively more asymmetrically wedge-shaped in three dimensions. As this occurs, flexibility is lost and rigidity increases. True lateral radiographs of the apical vertebra in mild, moderate, and severe curves demonstrate this beautifully (Fig. 3.26). If these asymmetrically wedged vertebrae were to be removed and given to the surgeon as pieces of blocks to stack as a column, they would not readily stack in any position other than that from which they were removed. Curve rigidity really means "unstackability": the greater the deformity, the more deformed the constituent vertebrae.

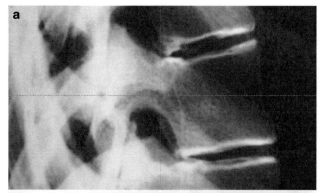

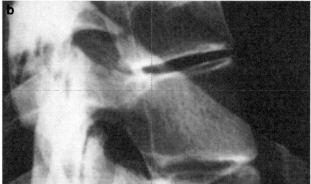

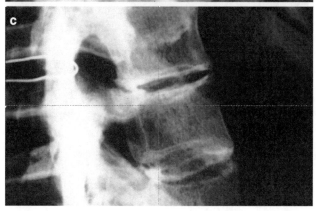

Fig. 3.26 True lateral radiographs of the apical vertebrae of idiopathic thoracic curves. (**a**) A mild curve. (**b**) A moderate curve. (**c**) A severe curve. With increasing curve magnitude the vertebrae are increasingly wedged in three dimensions so that the vertebral body endplates become less linear and more ellipsoid

This means that for curves over 60°, some additional maneuver is needed. For moderate 60–90° deformities, sufficient space for restacking can be achieved by performing multiple anterior discectomies over the apical five or six levels [40]. This allows the deformity to collapse into itself, so that not only is correction facilitated in the second stage but also the spine is not unduly lengthened in the process (Fig. 3.27). The second stage is the same posterior segmental instrumentation and fusion that would be performed as a one-stage procedure for a milder flexible curve. Such staged surgery is an important concept in scoliosis surgery and is key to achieving a safe and satisfactory correction.

There is a trend emerging of "two-in-one" surgery whereby both stages are performed under the same anesthetic. Proponents suggest that one long operation may have fewer complications than two shorter ones separated by a week or two. This may be so, but considerable deformity correction is often seen in the interval between operations, which may make the second posterior fusion safer. Spinal deformity surgery is very much a matter of risks and rewards, and while the rewards of a new and pleasing shape are considerable, risks should be kept to a minimum.

Early-Onset Idiopathic Scoliosis (Before 5 Years of Age)

Like progressive congenital scoliosis this can give rise to serious health problems such as cardiopulmonary compromise. Although the age divide for heart and lung troubles in later life is 5 years [7] the really worrying cases are the infantile idiopathic "malignant" progressive curves which, untreated, may exceed 100° in the first 2 years. The resulting disturbed alveolar reduplication can lead to severely hypoplastic lungs.

Clinical Features

Interestingly, when this condition was first reported from Holland by Harrenstein [41] the great majority of cases proved progressive, with only a minority resolving spontaneously. This state of affairs persisted for two or three decades. James [15] reported that only 4 of 33 cases resolved. The Oxford group reported that four times more progressed than resolved [42] but, for whatever reason, the proportions changed quite dramatically, and by the mid-1960s Lloyd-Roberts and Pilcher [43] reported 92 of 100 cases resolving. By 1968, only 5% progressed [44] and this remains the situation. In the 500 babies with early-onset idiopathic scoliosis we have treated in Yorkshire, we prescribe treatment in about 20%, in order to err on the safe side.

How is the deformity produced? One school of thought favors intrauterine and the other postnatal molding caused by the baby habitually lying in the oblique lateral decubitus position. There is more support for the latter theory as plagiocephaly develops only after birth. The "skew" baby with eccentric shape of head, thorax, and pelvis, together with unilateral bat ear, wryneck, and an adducted hip is linked to persistent sleeping on one side. There is also a greater incidence of mental retardation, congenital heart disease, inguinal hernia, breech delivery, low birth weight, older mothers, congenital hip dislocation, and familial predisposition [45].

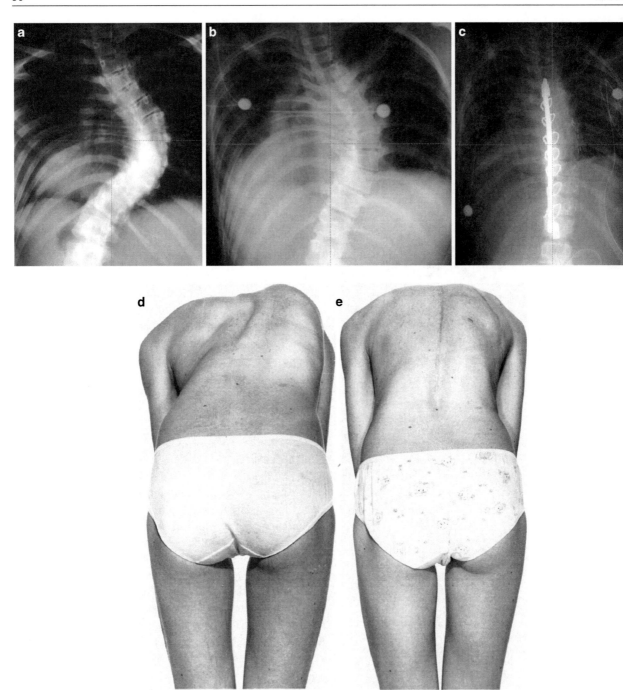

Fig. 3.27 Two-stage anterior and posterior corrections of a severe idiopathic thoracic curve. (**a**) PA radiograph showing a 90° right thoracic deformity. (**b**) PA radiograph in recovery just hours after anterior multiple discectomy. The deformity has lessened to a third of its original size simply by taking out five intervertebral discs and growth plates and allowing the leading edge to collapse. (**c**) PA radiograph a week later after posterior instrumentation showing an excellent correction of the deformity but more importantly an excellent correction of the chest wall asymmetry. (**d**) Forward-bending view before surgery showing a grotesque and rigid deformity. (**e**) Forward-bending view 6 months postoperatively showing a virtually complete correction in all planes

Males are affected more commonly than females, in a ration of 3:2, and thoracic curves are more common than thoraco-lumbar and double curve patterns. Most thoracic curves are to the left, and females with right-sided curves have a worse prognosis.

Mehta [46] described the rib vertebra angle difference (RVAD), recognizing it as a useful parameter in early-onset idiopathic scoliosis in helping to differentiate progressive from resolving scoliosis. On a PA radiograph of a thoracic curve the apical vertebra is located and its vertical axis drawn; lines are drawn along the necks of the associated ribs. The angles between these are the rib vertebra angles (RVAs), and when the smaller is subtracted from the larger the RVAD is calculated (Fig. 3.28). Mehta noted that when the RVAD exceeded 20° there was a significant risk of progression. The RVAD is probably a measure of the amount of rotation or torsion at the apex of the curve.

Some clinical factors are crucial in assessing these babies. A normal baby of 3.64 kg (8 lb), which reaches its milestones quickly, invariably has a mild deformity that will resolve. By contrast, a low birth weight, floppy, hypotonic baby which is slow to reach normal milestones has all the hallmarks of progression. Curve flexibility is important: this is best assessed by laying the baby gently over the examiner's knee, convex side downward, with the curve apex on the leg. If the shoulders and pelvis are allowed to sag, flexibility can be assessed. If the curve does not correct during this maneuver it is very likely to be progressive. These clinical and radiological evaluations ensure that no time is lost in managing the child with progressive deformity: curve deterioration can occur at an alarming rate.

Management

If the clinical and radiological evaluation suggests the likelihood of spontaneous resolution no treatment is required, but the child should be re-examined in 2–3 months. In the hypotonic, floppy, low birth weight baby treatment should start immediately, regardless of the radiological parameters. Borderline cases should also be dealt with as if they were progressive.

The only type of scoliosis that is really helped by nonoperative treatment is early-onset idiopathic scoliosis, for which serial elongation–de-rotation–flexion (EDF) casting is very successful [47]. The casts are applied under a light general anesthetic on a traction table and take advantage of the young, malleable skeleton. By exerting pressure on the convex ribs in an effort to untwist the spine while the plaster sets, one can achieve correction. The casts usually last for a period of 3 months before replacement. Such casts are surprisingly well tolerated by babies and mothers (Fig. 3.29).

If curve resolution occurs quickly, casting can be discontinued and observation maintained; otherwise serial casting should be continued until the age of 4 years, when infantile growth velocity has abated. At the pubertal growth spurt, careful observation is again important. Long-term follow-up has shown the remarkable success of EDF casting [48].

If curve progression continues despite casting or the patient presents with major deformity, operative treatment is required. This can be a daunting prospect as the very young spine is more cartilaginous than bony. These are lordoscolioses just like late-onset idiopathic curves and anterior overgrowth is the main driving force; posterior fusion is contraindicated and some form of instrumented "subcutaneous" spinal procedure is necessary. Lifting the periosteum

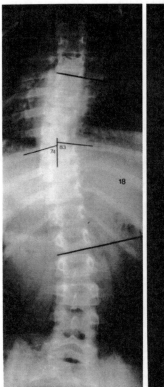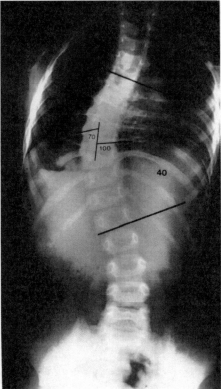

Fig. 3.28 The rib vertebra angle distance. (**a**) PA radiograph of an infantile idiopathic curve of 18° Cobb angle and only 9° rib RVAD. This might suggest a resolving curve but observe that the lumbar compensatory curve is indeed structural and, in particular, the 12th rib on the right side droops more than the left (a negative RVAD). This indicates that this is a double-structural curve and these have much greater progression potential than single curves. (**b**) PA radiograph of the same child a year later. He was not treated, the RVAD is now 30°, and the Cobb angle 40°. The double-structural curve pattern is more clearly visible

Fig. 3.29 (**a**) Applying an EDF cast for an infant with progressive infantile idiopathic scoliosis. An hour well spent. (**b**) PA radiograph of a boy of 4 years at presentation to the scoliosis clinic showing a thoracic deformity in excess of 100°. In the radiograph packet there was a film taken 2 years earlier showing a deformity of only 30°. Urgent referral and treatment is essential

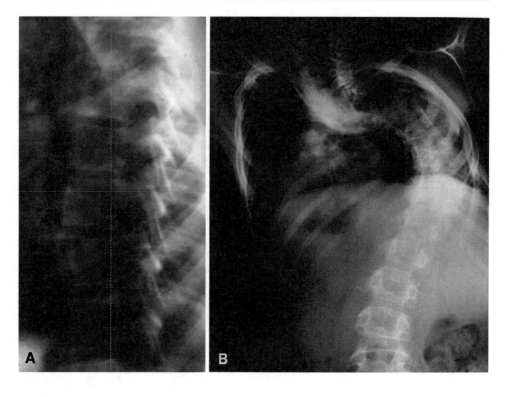

might produce osteogenesis and so, although the hooks at top and bottom will be subperiosteal, the intervening rod must be extraperiosteal [49]. It may be possible to manage the child throughout skeletal growth with posterior subcutaneous instrumentation, extending or replacing the rod as necessary. However, anterior growth ablation is often required by anterior discectomy and removal of the growth plates over the middle one-third to two-fifths of the curve to control anterior overgrowth.

This gives rise to an anterior fusion over the operated segments but leaves several segments above and below the subcutaneous rod for growth throughout childhood (Fig. 3.30) until definitive posterior spinal fusion is necessary if it does not occur spontaneously.

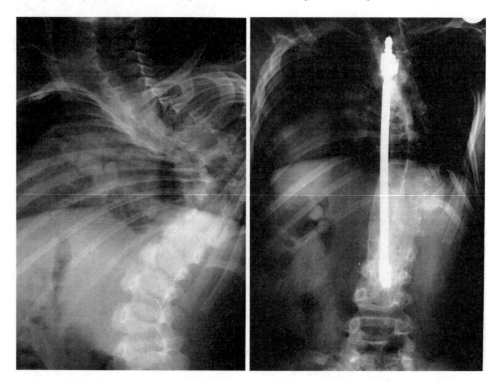

Fig. 3.30 (**a**) PA radiograph of a severe infantile idiopathic progressive thoracic scoliosis in a boy aged 5 years, despite EDF casting. (**b**) PA radiograph 10 years after anterior growth ablation over the apical region and 10 posterior growing rod lengthenings/replacements. An excellent correction has been achieved. A posterior fusion has spontaneously developed

Newer generation metalwork systems have been developed in which one or two longitudinal rods are connected with a domino in the middle. By loosening the domino, distracting, and retightening, the construct can be lengthened with growth.

Roaf in 1963 [50] tried to control the growth of early-onset idiopathic curves by an antero-convex hemiepiphysiodesis. Unfortunately, while this worked for coronal plane deformities such as a solid hemivertebra, it did not work for the rotational lordoscoliosis of infantile idiopathic scoliosis [51]. Epiphysiodesis may alter growth but cannot counter the unfavorable buckling biomechanics of the underlying lordosis.

Recently there has been a resurgence of interest in restraining growth on the antero-convex side of the spine by stapling but no long-term results are available. Elevating the periosteum may not be as osteogenic as is generally believed, and the Luque segmental wire fixation system may be an option for posterior metalwork: as the back of the spine grows, the wires can migrate down the L-rods (the "Luque trolley") [1]. It also allows the correction to occur in kyphosis rather than lordosis (Fig. 3.31).

To avoid tackling the spine in severe deformity, the ribs have recently been the target of instrumentation with the vertical expandable prosthetic titanium rib procedure (VEPTR) [52] (Fig. 3.32). These need regular replacement surgically and long-term results are not yet available.

With EDF casting most scolioses either resolve or can be held relatively static until the adolescent growth spurt; management then is similar to late-onset idiopathic scoliosis. For those that resolve, it is the rotational component that may take several years to untwist, long after the spine appears straight on the AP radiograph.

Idiopathic Hyperkyphosis (Scheuermann's Disease)

Type I thoracic Scheuermann's disease is the opposite condition to idiopathic thoracic scoliosis (Figs. 3.10b and 3.33). It tends to occur in males and, although it has a community prevalence and familial trend similar to idiopathic

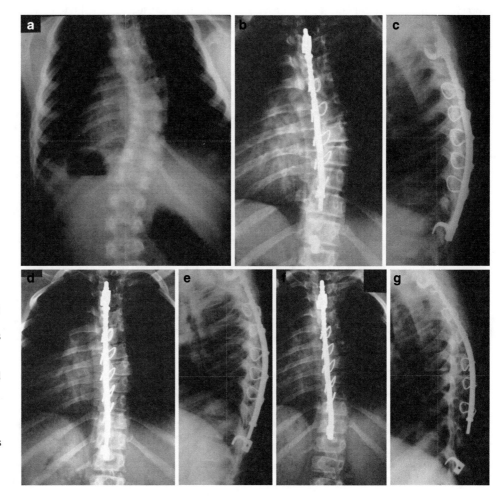

Fig. 3.31 Harrington–Luque trolley. (**a**) PA radiograph of a 5-year old whose curve could not be controlled by EDF casting. (**b**) PA and (**c**) lateral radiographs after recreation of the thoracic kyphosis using a Harrington rod and sublaminar wires. (**d**) PA and (**e**) lateral radiographs 3 years later showing that the lower end of the rod has almost grown out of the lower hook. (**f**) PA and (**g**) lateral radiographs taken 10 years later show that the spine has remained corrected and grown more than 2 inches

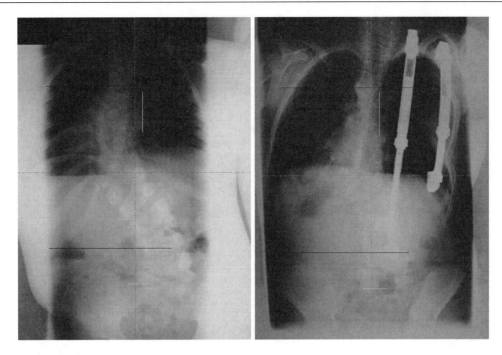

Fig. 3.32 (**a**) PA radiograph of a progressive early-onset case. (**b**) PA radiograph after insertion of the VEPTR apparatus to distract the ribs on the concave side

thoracic scoliosis, it has a later age of onset: most patients present about 2 years before skeletal maturity [12]. The condition is frequently painful, although the pain is usually fatigue discomfort over the lower part of the kyphosis, rather than significant night pain, is suggestive of a more

sinister lesion. Patients present with either increasing thoracic round back, pain, or both. Unlike the benign postural round back deformity, which is fully flexible on extension, type I Scheuermann's disease is characteristically rigid: on forward bending there is an angular apex to the kyphosis

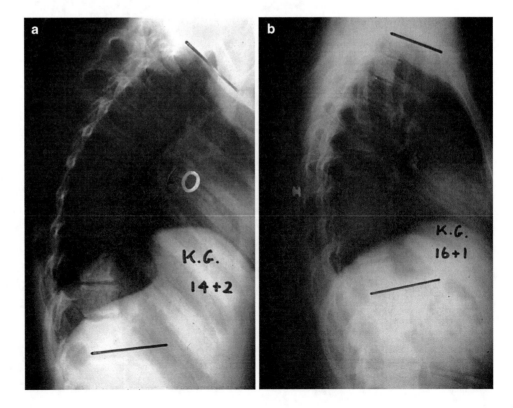

Fig. 3.33 (**a**) Lateral radiograph of a boy with a 60° thoracic Scheuermann's kyphosis. (**b**) After extension bracing 2 years later a normal kyphosis has been restored

rather than the smooth hyperkyphosis of the postural round back deformity. Pressure on this angular apex demonstrates its rigidity. Pectus carinatum or other deformity of the anterior chest wall is common and becomes more obvious with larger kyphoses. There is also characteristic and considerable hamstring tightness. Lower-limb neurological abnormalities are rare and occur only with very severe angular deformity when the spinal cord is tightly stretched. Two-thirds have a mild idiopathic scoliosis below the hyperkyphosis (Fig. 3.11).

Lateral radiographs of the spine show vertebral wedging with a reduced anterior versus posterior height. There is often evidence of anterior Schmorl node formation or endplate irregularity (Fig. 3.10b). The AP view may show a slight scoliosis with no rotation in the region of the kyphosis if the anterior growth plate is affected asymmetrically.

Unlike idiopathic thoracic scoliosis, thoracic Scheuermann's disease is treatable conservatively, provided the spine is not too kyphotic and that some spinal growth remains. Because the deformity exists in the sagittal plane and is rotationally stable, extension bracing or casting generally restores an acceptable sagittal profile within a year or so (Fig. 3.33). This should then be followed by extension exercises until spinal maturity is reached in the early to mid-twenties. Even if a patient is beyond general skeletal maturity worthwhile improvement may follow conservative management by extension.

For severe deformities correction can be achieved only by operation. Even with extensive surgery only a 40% correction is possible and not without risk to the patient. Although two-stage anterior multiple discectomy and interbody grafting followed by posterior segmental instrumentation is favored, it is possible to achieve a reasonable correction by posterior surgery alone. The pseudarthrosis rate, however, is much greater than in idiopathic scoliosis, because the posterior fusion is on the tension side of the kyphosis. In the balance between risks and rewards, the rewards are less obvious than in idiopathic thoracic scoliosis.

With the exceptional case of neurological dysfunction in the lower limbs, confirmed by imaging as due to the angular hyperkyphosis, the only satisfactory surgical solution is anterior dural decompression by apical vertebral body resection and anterior strut grafting.

Type II Scheuermann's disease, "apprentice's spine" (Fig. 3.34), nearly always presents as local thoraco-lumbar pain rather than deformity. However, sometimes patients present with mechanical low back pain because of the high prevalence of associated lower lumbar spondylolyses, which may be multiple. As the hypertrophic callus around these lyses can irritate local nerve roots, a careful history and neurological examination of the lower extremities are essential. The radiographs should also include oblique views of the lower lumbar spine to search for lyses. The pain of type II

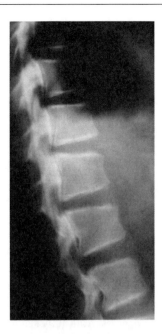

Fig. 3.34 Lateral thoraco-lumbar myelogram showing thoraco-lumbar type 2 Scheuermann's disease with significant vertebral body kyphotic wedging. There were intermittent neurological symptoms but no myelographic abnormality

Scheuermann's disease generally settles with conservative measures, which may include rest in a spinal support.

Congenital Deformities

Congenital deformities of the spine comprise two basic types—congenital bone deformities and congenital spinal cord deformities—although coexistence is common. Congenital spinal cord deformities are those of spina bifida and myelodysplasia (see Chapter 4 of Children's Neuromuscular Disorders), whereas congenital bony deformities are failures of vertebral formation or segmentation. Embryologically, mesenchyme migrates to surround the notochord; a breakdown of the medial surface of the somites leads to bony deformities. The segmental pattern of sclerotomal mesenchyme is staggered relative to the part of the somite left behind, so forming segmental muscle blocks. As a result the spinal nerves and muscles are segmental, whereas the vertebrae are intersegmental.

The re-segmentation theory was formulated to explain this complex, staggered arrangement, but this has been challenged by Verbout [53], who demonstrated clearly that all the elements of the future vertebral column develop in their definitive positions and that re-segmentation was neither required nor occurred. In any event, as early as the fourth week of intrauterine life, spinal structure and shape are developing and interference with this delicate process results in a variety of congenital spinal deformities.

Congenital Bony Deformities

Congenital bony deformities derive either from failures of formation or from failures of segmentation (Fig. 3.35); both probably relate to abnormalities of the intersegmental arteries leading to abnormal differential growth of mesenchymal cells at different sites in the developing spinal column—i.e., lateral, anterior, posterior, or at disc level. Lateral defects produce scoliosis, anterior defects kyphosis, and posterior defects lordosis, but defects commonly exist in at least two planes, producing a three-dimensional deformity.

Failures of Formation

Failures of formation are either wedge-shaped vertebrae or hemivertebrae. Furthermore, the hemivertebra can be segmented to varying degrees, from fully segmented (with disc spaces and growth plates both above and below) to nonsegmented (no disc space or growth plates above and below and the vertebra effectively fused to its adjacent neighbors). In simple terms, the more growth available, the more significant the potential deformity: the fully segmented hemivertebra is more likely to produce a progressive deformity than the non-segmented variety (Fig. 3.35). Nonetheless, even a fully segmented solitary hemivertebra generally has a benign prognosis. It tends to exist in the coronal plane and produces a lateral scoliosis with no significant rotation and generally requires observation only. However, in the lumbosacral region, a solitary hemivertebra with an oblique lumbosacral

takeoff can produce an ugly and progressive list of the trunk (Fig. 3.36). Of course, when double or multiple hemivertebrae occur on the same side, progressive and unacceptable deformities may develop.

In the sagittal plane, dorsal hemivertebrae produce progressive angular kyphoses. With growth, the hemivertebra can be squeezed out posteriorly into the front of the spinal canal and lead to impending paraplegia with hyperreflexia and clonus. Careful follow-up with neurological assessment is essential.

Failures of Segmentation

Failures of segmentation mean that one or more adjacent vertebrae fail to develop normal discs and growth plates. Complete failure of segmentation gives rise to a block vertebra—adjacent vertebrae with no disc space between. These are often found as routine radiological anomalies in otherwise healthy individuals. Partial failures of segmentation, with discs and growth plates on one side only of the spine (unilateral bars), progress more aggressively than their failure of formation counterparts. There are two reasons for this: first there is no growth on the other side, so that progression is the rule; second, unilateral bars in the coronal plane tend to involve the sagittal plane with a lordosis and thus superimpose a biomechanical buckling akin to idiopathic scoliosis. Indeed, such patients can present with a similar rotational prominence, and only the radiograph

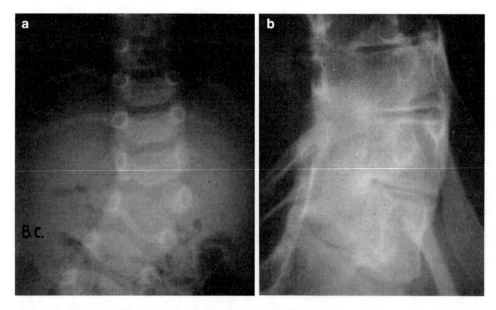

Fig. 3.35 (**a**) PA radiograph showing a hemivertebra (unilateral failure of formation). This is well segmented with growth plates above and below. A progressive deformity can develop. (**b**) PA radiograph showing a unilateral bar (unilateral failure of segmentation) extending over four vertebrae. There is no growth on the concave side and so a progressive deformity of significance will develop

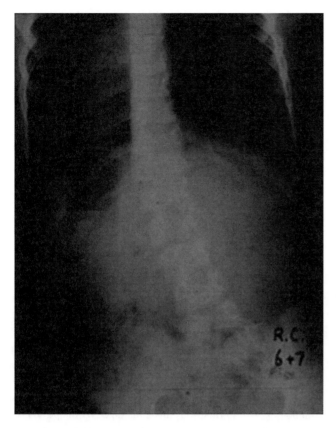

Fig. 3.36 PA radiograph of a lumbar spine showing a lumbosacral hemivertebra producing a marked torso list

demonstrates the underlying congenital deformity. A particularly sinister combination is a unilateral bar on one side with a hemivertebra on the other: inexorable progression is the rule.

Failures of segmentation also occur in the sagittal plane: an anterior bar causes progressive kyphosis but, unlike a dorsal hemivertebra, which is squeezed into the spinal canal, neurological problems are rare. Patients present with progressive deformity, which tends to be less angular and less severe than that caused by a dorsal hemivertebra.

Treatment

If the child is referred to the orthopaedic surgeon by a paediatrician, systems other than the locomotor system have usually already been assessed. If, however, the orthopaedic surgeon is the first examiner, he must organize appropriate investigations, including abdominal ultrasound to assess the renal tract (there is a high incidence of congenital urological malformations in association with congenital spinal anomalies). In addition, the full length of the spine should be evaluated by radiograph, MRI, and/or computed tomography (CT) myelography because of the high incidence of

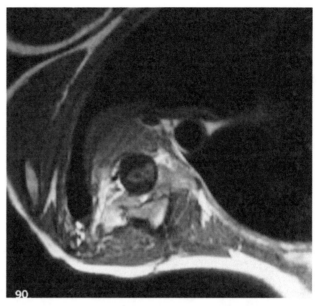

Fig. 3.37 Axial MRI slice showing two spinal cords split by a diastematomyelia

spinal dysraphism (Fig. 3.37). In spinal dysraphism, however, the spine column is never normal on plain films: there is widening of the interpedicular distance at the level of the diastematomyelia (midline bony or fibrous spur cleaving the spinal cord sagittally). A diastematomyelia or a low conus secondary to a tethered filum must be excluded before operation to avoid tension paralysis (a tight filum may need division or a diastematomyelia excision before tackling the spinal deformity).

As with idiopathic scoliosis, conservative treatment is of no value: treatment is surgical for both scoliosis and kyphosis. The general indications for operation are similar to those for idiopathic scoliosis. Significant deformities of early onset require treatment to mitigate against subsequent cardiopulmonary problems; later-onset deformities are more a question of appearance than of function. The anomaly associated with the most severe progression—the unilateral bar on one side with a failure of formation on the other—is sufficiently sinister to consider early prophylactic fusion. This is easier said than done; posterior fusion may make matters worse by tethering the back of the spine. Logic suggests a combined anterior and posterior fusion, but this is a formidable undertaking, particularly in the young cartilaginous spine and no published evidence testifies to its prophylactic benefit. Indeed, despite prophylactic anterior and posterior fusions, the deformity may progress inexorably, presumably as the result of plastic deformation of the fusion mass from biomechanical buckling. Furthermore, if anterior and posterior prophylactic fusions fail to halt progression, subsequent corrective surgery is made difficult or even impossible because of pleural adhesions from previous surgery.

Moreover, the natural history of congenital scoliosis is not always predictable and not all potentially serious growth asymmetries produce unacceptable deformities. When definite progression does occur operation should be advised to avoid irreversible chest problems. Otherwise it is sensible to review regularly as all anomalies do lead to unacceptable deformity [54].

When deformity is unacceptable the only safe way to alter spinal shape significantly is by two-stage wedge resection of the curve apex, so that correction is not accompanied by tension lengthening of the spinal cord. Roaf's concept of antero-convex hemiepiphysiodesis was sound biologically but is only reliable for the solitary hemivertebra, which seldom progresses to unacceptability [50]. It is ineffective for failures of segmentation as the underlying lordotic deformity has driven further deformity before the biological effect of epiphysiodesis can occur with growth [51]. Leatherman and Dickson [55] concluded that it is better to wait for the deformity to declare itself and to carry out a two-stage closing wedge resection once serious progression has taken place. Removing the apical keystone vertebra (Fig. 3.38) with prophylactic anterior fusion of the levels above and below is a much more certain way of controlling asymmetric spinal growth at a young age than prophylactic fusion. Isolated removal of a hemivertebra is usually only indicated for a lumbosacral hemivertebra causing progressive imbalance and trunk list. At other sites, prophylactic posterior fusion at an earlier stage may be preferable to hemivertebra excision to reduce the risk of cord dysfunction.

Congenital kyphosis needs surgical treatment if any abnormal neurological signs develop in the lower limbs.

Operation entails anterior dural decompression by excision of the dorsal hemivertebra, interbody strut grafting, and posterior instrumental support.

Congenital Spinal Cord Deformities

This refers to the spina bifida syndromes (see Chapter 4 of Children's Neuromuscular Disorders). More significant myelodysplasia is linked with more severe spinal deformity: patients with total neurological loss in the lower extremities are most likely to develop the most severe deformities. The majority of these are long C-shaped paralytic lordoscolioses with pelvic obliquity (Fig. 3.39).

Progressive trunk imbalance imperils walking and sitting, and undue pressure on the lower buttock may produce recurrent pressure sores with serious even life-threatening effects. These are difficult deformities to manage: the extensive anterior and posterior surgery necessary has a high complication rate and the risk/benefit equation needs careful evaluation.

For those with sufficient lower-limb function to walk, spinal surgery is contraindicated because a rigid lumbar spine can send them off their feet and make them permanent wheelchair users. Some patients who are wheelchair sitters with no lower-limb function can be managed by the provision of a total contact "Derby" seat in their wheelchair. However, for the patient with a progressive trunk list compelled to use upper limbs for support in the wheelchair, surgical correction and fusion are indicated.

The objective is to provide a square pelvis with a balanced spine above. This requires anterior and posterior instrumentation and fusion down to the sacrum. Anterior segmental instrumentation is favored for the first stage and posterior

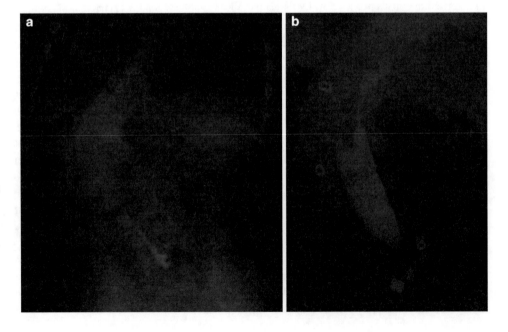

Fig. 3.38 Wedge resection for a severe congenital spinal deformity. (**a**) PA radiograph of an 8-year-old girl with a 95° rigid thoraco-lumbar scoliosis. (**b**) Preoperative myelogram demonstrating a split spinal cord due to a diastematomyelia. (**c**) PA radiograph after two-stage wedge resection showing an excellent correction. During the second posterior stage the diastematomyelia was removed

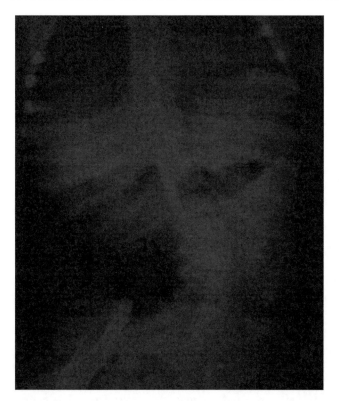

Fig. 3.39 PA radiograph of a spina bifida patient showing the typical C-shaped thoraco-lumbar deformity with severe pelvic obliquity

instrumentation for the second. This must vary in accordance with the local anatomy. Areas with wide posterior element deficiency can be managed by transpedicular instrumentation but the spine above can be dealt with by hooks or segmental wires.

Careful preoperative assessment is important as up to 40% of patients with paralytic lordoscolioses also have a significant congenital bony anomaly (e.g., a hemivertebra or bar) in the thoraco-lumbar region above the spina bifida that can produce torso imbalance (Fig. 3.40).

Some severely affected children also have a congenital deficiency of the anterior spinal column in the lumbar region and develop progressive lumbar kyphoses. They are eventually drawn so far forward that the anterior chest wall rests on the anterior thighs (Fig. 3.41). All the anterior structures, even the anterior abdominal wall, contract secondarily and may need to be surgically released if the deformity is to be effectively straightened.

Congenital Spinal Deformity Syndromes

Congenital spinal deformities are encountered in a number of generalized conditions such as Goldenhar's syndrome (hemifacial dysplasia), Treacher-Collins syndrome

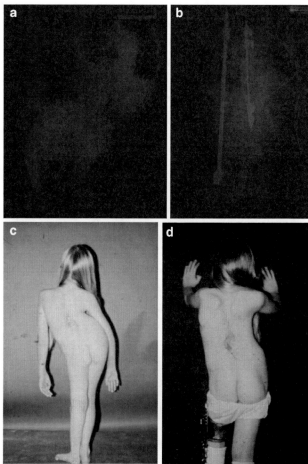

Fig. 3.40 (**a**) PA radiograph of a spina bifida patient with a congenital bony failure of segmentation in the thoracic spine above posterior element deficiency in the lumbar spine and a significantly tilted pelvis. The pelvic tilt is caused principally by the upper congenital bony deformity decompensating the spine. There was also a shortened, weakened, and attenuated left lower extremity. (**b**) After two-stage wedge resection of the upper congenital bony anomaly and then posterior instrumentation extending down to the pelvis, an excellent correction has been achieved. Note the old Harrington instrumentation as most scoliosis clinics have not seen a spina bifida patient for two or three decades. (**c**) Posterior view of this patient who was "going off her feet." (**d**) Postoperative view of this patient. Surgery put her back into balance although she required a knee brace and foot raise for the left lower extremity

(mandibulo-facial dysostosis), Crouzon's syndrome (craniofacial dysostosis), Apert's syndrome (craniofacial dysostosis plus syndactyly), and Larsen's syndrome (multiple congenital dislocations with a characteristic facies). Progressive deformities are not uncommon in these children but other major clinical considerations may take precedence over the spinal deformity.

Klippel–Feil syndrome incorporates congenital bony anomalies in the cervico-thoracic region with a short neck, low hairline, and restricted cervical movement (Fig. 3.42; see Chapter 1). Progressive deformity, associated wryneck, facial asymmetry, and Sprengel's shoulder (see Chapter 2 of Children's Upper and Lower Limb Orthopaedic Disorders)

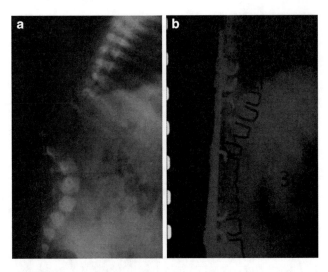

Fig. 3.41 The congenital kyphosis of myelomeningocele. (**a**) Preoperative lateral radiograph. (**b**) Lateral radiograph 5 years after radical anterior soft tissue release and discectomy followed by posterior instrumentation; sitting stability has been restored

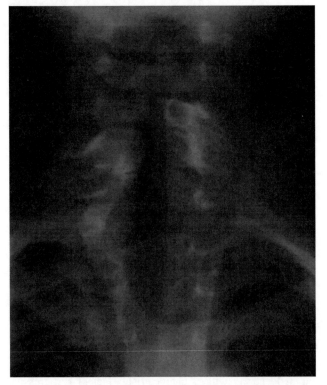

Fig. 3.42 PA radiograph of the cervico-thoracic region showing the typical multiple congenital abnormalities of Klippel–Feil syndrome

can produce a very unfavorable appearance, but corrective surgery in the cervico-thoracic region is difficult, dangerous, and not recommended. Congenital intervertebral fusions reduce the number of motion segments and the resulting

instability particularly in the upper cervical spine may lead to neurological problems. Limited simple fusion then has an important role.

In the lumbosacral spine the bony skeleton may completely or partially fail to form resulting in lumbosacral agenesis. With complete lumbar absence, the appearance is that of a "sitting Buddha"; however, more often, the lesions are partial. Many patients have significant urogenital or alimentary tract problems, which override the spine in priority, but for those with spino-pelvic instability, fusion may be necessary.

Other Spinal Deformities

Neuromuscular Deformities

The true neuromuscular diseases of childhood are those which affect the spinal cord, peripheral nerves, neuromuscular junctions, and muscles [56]. They include spinal muscular atrophy, the peripheral neuropathies, Friedreich's ataxia, arthrogryposis, and the muscular dystrophies. It is convenient also to include in this section cerebral palsy and poliomyelitis.

The common denominator is the spinal column buckling associated with inadequate neuromuscular control. Not surprisingly, the most severe neuromuscular problems usually cause the most severe progressive spinal deformities. Thus, in cerebral palsy those at the milder end of the spectrum, with minimal brain dysfunction, may develop no spinal deformity, whereas those with total body involvement almost invariably develop a significant scoliosis. In general two types of scoliosis are encountered:

1. An idiopathic-type deformity above a square and stable pelvis.
2. A collapsing C-shaped lordoscoliosis associated with the more severe forms of paralysis.

The idiopathic-type curves above a stable pelvis tend to appear in less-affected individuals, whereas the collapsing paralytic curves are more prevalent in those more severely affected.

Management of the spinal deformity must not be considered in isolation: it is essential to assess the whole patient. Nevertheless broad therapeutic generalizations can be made accepting that they may sometimes need radical changes.

Patients with a mild neuromuscular problem and idiopathic-type curves above a stable pelvis can be treated like those with idiopathic scoliosis. Patients with collapsing paralytic deformities with pelvic obliquity must to be assessed with regard to function rather than shape. If the patient is a walker, surgical treatment is contraindicated because interference with a mobile lumbar lordosis can stop walking and render the patient wheelchair-bound. However, as many deformities prove progressive and walking ability is lost, surgery if necessary can then be undertaken. When, to achieve wheelchair stability, the patient needs upper limbs for support the arms cannot be used for other purposes and corrective spinal surgery is functionally very helpful.

Many collapsing paralytic scolioses remain remarkably flexible despite their size in the sitting position. Most can therefore be dealt with by posterior instrumentation. Although two-rod systems using transpedicular metalwork have become popular, sublaminar wiring to L-rods is still an acceptable option (Fig. 3.43).

Cerebral Palsy

Considerable judgment is required to assess whether a patient with a seemingly treatable deformity has the overall ability to complete safely and successfully a difficult and lengthy treatment program. Even in specialized centers complications are the rule rather than the exception. Although lost function is the prime indicator for operation, only a minority of patients demonstrate improved function. Probably, only those who are losing sitting stability should be treated surgically [57] (Fig. 3.44).

Poliomyelitis

After the convalescent phase, when recovery can still occur, the residual deformities can be widespread and may include scoliosis and pelvic obliquity. Understanding the causes

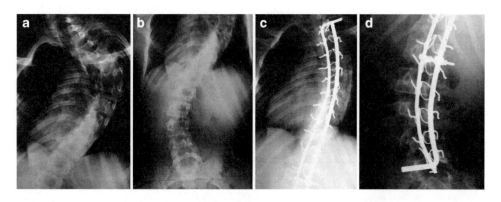

Fig. 3.43 (**a** and **b**) Preoperative supine radiographs of a wheelchair-bound teenager with Friedreich's ataxia. He was losing sitting stability. (**c** and **d**) Postoperative PA radiographs following Luque sublaminar wiring

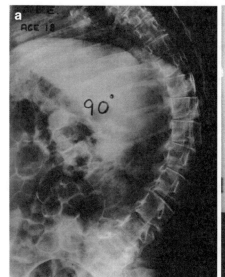
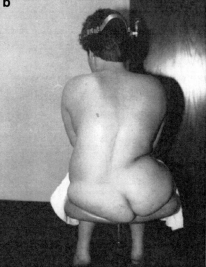
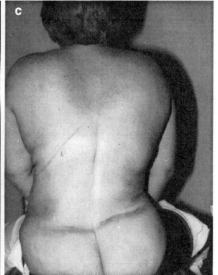

Fig. 3.44 (**a**) PA radiograph of a severe scoliosis with pelvic obliquity in an 18-year-old boy with cerebral palsy. He was bed-bound and in no pain. There was no indication for treatment. (**b**) Preoperative back view of a young teenage girl with a scoliosis and severe pelvic obliquity threatening sitting stability. (**c**) Back view 5 years after anterior and posterior instrumentation and fusion. Sitting stability has been restored

of pelvic obliquity is important in assessing spinal deformity. There are three types: infrapelvic, suprapelvic, and transpelvic. Lower-limb length inequality or contracture cause *infrapelvic* obliquity; loss of trunk balance due to scoliosis causes *suprapelvic* obliquity and unequal contracture of the ilio-psoas muscles (which alone span the pelvis) causes *transpelvic* obliquity. Suprapelvic obliquity is much underrated: it is fruitless trying to prevent progressive hip subluxation by hip surgery in the presence of suprapelvic obliquity rather than by correcting and stabilizing the scoliosis. This reduces the pelvic obliquity and improves femoral head cover. As with other non-spastic neuromuscular disorders, the scoliosis of poliomyelitis is usually flexible and can be treated by powerful posterior segmental instrumentation and fusion.

Spinal Muscular Atrophy

This was previously subdivided into the early-onset Werdnig–Hoffmann and later-onset Kugelberg-Welander varieties but is better regarded as a continuum with severe, intermediate, and mild subgroups [58]. The severe infantile onset group dies within 2 years and orthopaedic treatment addresses only the intermediate and mild groups. This is an anterior horn cell problem and electromyography and muscle biopsy are required to differentiate it from the Becker or limb girdle dystrophies (see Chapter 3 of Children's Neuromuscular Disorders).

Although walking may be possible for many years, patients who live long enough become confined to a wheelchair. Again, spinal surgery should not be undertaken too early as it can impair walking ability. Many patients develop contractures of the lower limbs and around the hips, compounding the scoliosis and pelvic obliquity. If surgery is considered for the collapsing spine of a sitting patient, chest function may be the limiting factor: some degree of postoperative atelectasis or chest infection occurs in most patients and several days of endotracheal intubation or even preoperative tracheotomy are often necessary. Although the heart is not involved, reduced pulmonary function contraindicates operating via the diaphragm. The prime candidate for scoliosis surgery is the patient with a relatively flexible deformity that can be handled by posterior segmental instrumentation only [59].

Peripheral Neuropathies, Friedreich's Ataxia, and Arthrogryposis

Orthopaedic surgeons often encounter and first diagnose these patients. Pes cavus and a high-stepping gait typify the hereditary sensorimotor neuropathies, and a broad-based ataxic gait suggests Friedreich's ataxia. Cardiomyopathy is associated with Friedreich's ataxia and some forms of hypertrophic polyneuritis are also linked with heart problems [56]. Anterior spinal surgery should be avoided and it is important that affected children should undergo careful paediatric scrutiny before considering posterior segmental instrumentation and fusion (Fig. 3.43). The more rigid curves that sometimes occur in some forms of arthrogryposis require two-stage anterior and posterior instrumentation.

The Muscular Dystrophies

Patients with the milder Becker, limb girdle, and facio-scapulo-humeral varieties of muscular dystrophy tolerate scoliosis operations well, but those with Duchenne dystrophy or congenital myopathies, although they may benefit the most, are at much greater risk (see Chapter 3 of Children's Neuromuscular Disorders). Anterior surgery is contraindicated because of the associated cardiomyopathy. One-stage posterior segmental instrumentation and fusion should be undertaken when these unfortunate patients lose walking ability because the inevitable progressive spinal deformation can be successfully prevented while they are in their best physical condition. Surgery is hazardous because of the cardiomyopathy and the tendency to excessive bleeding. Surgeons performing this type of surgery have to accept a mortality rate as high as 10% [60].

Deformities Associated with Von Recklinghausen's Disease

Neurofibromatosis (type NF-1) involves many tissues of the body—cutaneous, subcutaneous, nervous, skeletal, vascular, and lymphatic. Although an autosomal dominant, more than 50% of cases are new mutations. Any two of the following features are considered diagnostic:

- a positive family history
- a positive nodule biopsy
- six café au lait spots
- the presence of multiple nodules

As with many inherited conditions it is not so much the condition that matters as its individual severity of expression. Scoliosis is the most common skeletal manifestation, developing in almost 50% of patients. Its prevalence, progression potential, and the age of the child at onset are proportional to the degree of dystrophic bone change (Fig. 3.45) [61]. Thus attenuated "penciled" ribs, enlarged intervertebral foraminae, and vertebral scalloping are associated with early-onset curves with significant potential for progression. Moreover,

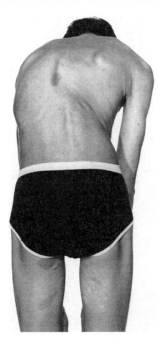

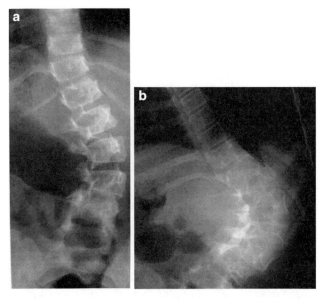

Fig. 3.46 (**a**) PA radiograph of the lumbar spine of a child with a typical dystrophic Von Recklinghausen curve. Unfortunately no treatment was offered. (**b**) PA radiograph 2 years later. Do not delay with Von Recklinghausen dystrophic curves

Fig. 3.45 The typical appearance of a boy with Von Recklinghausen's disease. There are multiple café au lait skin patches and a short sharp angular thoraco-lumbar curve with rotation

such curves are typically short, sharp, and angular with a lot of apical rotation. By contrast, less dystrophic bone change makes scoliosis less prevalent, and, if it occurs, less severe: the curves resemble straightforward idiopathic scoliosis.

Reports of patients with Von Recklinghausen's scoliosis frequently and erroneously call the deformity kyphoscoliosis. While these short, sharp, angular dystrophic curves can *look* kyphotic, with a posterior chest wall prominence on the convex side, the apical vertebral bodies are found immediately under the convex ribs: the front of the spine points backward or, in more simple terms, the lordosis has buckled all the way round, so that it now effectively points posteriorly (Fig. 3.45).

As with idiopathic and congenital scoliosis, the earlier the onset and the greater the progression potential, the more difficult it is to obtain a lasting correction. The Von Recklinghausen's curve is notorious, as bone graft is often rapidly resorbed rather than consolidated. A golden rule is that the dystrophic curve always requires anterior and posterior fusions with excision of the anterior growth plates. If the curve is acceptable, then early anterior and posterior fusions are required. If the deformity is unacceptable, less severe curves can be dealt with by anterior multiple discectomies, followed by posterior instrumentation and fusion. The most severe curves require wedge resection.

At the milder end of the spectrum, these deformities can be managed like their idiopathic counterparts, but if the patient is young and features suggest dystrophic change, an anterior stage should be performed.

Pure kyphoses, akin to early-onset severe angular Scheuermann's kyphosis, are much less common than scolioses but can produce progressive lower-limb paralysis. They should be treated by anterior decompression and strut grafting.

Cervical spine deformities are not uncommon in Von Recklinghausen's disease and can be extremely complex, with an area of lordoscoliosis at one level and angular kyphosis at another. Again, anterior and posterior fusions are necessary, although access can be difficult.

Heritable Disorders of Connective Tissue, Mucopolysaccharidoses, and Skeletal Dysplasias

About 70% of patients with osteogenesis imperfecta (see Chapter 6 of General Principles of Children's Orthopaedic Disease) develop a scoliosis (Fig. 3.47) [62]. Even in those who do not the spine is abnormal with changes similar to juvenile osteoporosis (multiple compression fractures and biconcave vertebrae). Patients with spinal deformity are nearly always those with severe disease. Like Von Recklinghausen's disease, the more dystrophic the bone the earlier the onset and the more progressive the spinal deformity. Because of the problems of bone quality and strength in relationship to instrumentation it has been said that progressive curves require stabilization or nothing. To spread the load segmental instrumentation is preferred. Adding

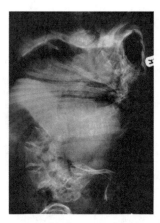

Fig. 3.47 PA radiograph of the spine in severe osteogenesis imperfecta. The main deformity is a huge right thoracic curve

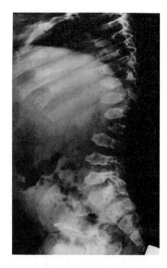

Fig. 3.48 Lateral radiograph of the thoraco-lumbar spine in a patient with Morquio's syndrome showing the typical platyspondyly and apical bullet-shaped vertebra

methyl methacrylate cement to hook sites merely moves the weakness problem to another interface. The improved bone density following bisphosphonate treatment may make spinal surgery less hazardous.

Marfan's syndrome, homocystinuria, congenital contractural arachnodactyly, Ehlers–Danlos syndrome, and their various formes frustes, are all associated with a greater prevalence rate of the idiopathic type of scoliosis as the spinal column is disadvantaged at the soft tissue level by these inherited disorders of ligamentous laxity [63]. The resulting deformities should be dealt with like their idiopathic counterparts. The patient with Marfan's syndrome may have significant heart valve and aortic disease, but this seldom presents a problem in adolescent scoliosis surgery. With homocystinuria, however, vascular damage may lead to thrombosis and it is important to avoid unnecessary surgery in these patients. Similarly, it is important to differentiate the various types of Ehlers–Danlos syndrome, in order to avoid surgery in those with vascular fragility, in whom excessive bleeding is a serious problem.

Of the mucopolysaccharidoses, MPS4 (Morquio's syndrome) is the most important to the spinal surgeon because of its two common and major spinal problems—thoraco-lumbar kyphosis and atlanto-axial instability. The thoraco-lumbar kyphosis is associated with platyspondyly and the apical anteriorly beaked vertebra may gradually produce cord compression (Fig. 3.48). There is some evidence that an extension trunk brace can be helpful but once neurological signs develop anterior decompression becomes necessary.

Atlanto-axial instability results from a deficient odontoid and this is a significant source of mortality and neurological morbidity [64]. It is common also in the spondyloepiphyseal dysplasias. Untreated, most patients develop myelopathy. Thus C1–C2 fusion is generally recommended prophylactically in all cases by the age of 10 years. This can be performed posteriorly, with a supportive halo-vest.

Achondroplasia

There are two important spinal problems that occur in these patients: thoraco-lumbar kyphosis and spinal stenosis [65]. Spinal stenosis, which tends to be more marked lower down the spine, is a problem of late adolescence and early adulthood and presents with claudication in the leg, weakness related to exercise, and gradually increasing neurological abnormalities in the legs. MRI confirms the diagnosis and decompressive laminectomy is required to prevent progressive paralysis and aid recovery. If this is performed on the immature spine, it is important to add a concomitant fusion to prevent progressive kyphosis (see Fig. 2.2).

Thoraco-lumbar kyphosis is a constant feature of achondroplasia, with a bullet-shaped apical vertebra. Seventy-five percent of these kyphoses resolve with growth, and treatment is only indicated if there are signs of impending paralysis. Occasionally there can be occipitalization of C1 with stenosis of the foramen magnum and secondary atlanto-axial instability: posterior C1–C2 fusion is then indicated.

Other Dysplasias

Spondyloepiphyseal dysplasia can also be associated with a thoraco-lumbar bullet-shaped vertebra, but posterior vertebral humping differentiates this from Morquio's syndrome. Kyphosis akin to Scheuermann's disease can also occur and is amenable to extension bracing, but if the bullet-shaped vertebra produces impending paralysis anterior cord decompression and grafting are required.

Scoliosis is not uncommon in diastrophic dysplasia and, again, the dystrophic bone favors buckling and anterior and posterior fusions are necessary. A particularly nasty deformity in this condition is cervical kyphosis. These patients require careful neurological monitoring and any tendency toward progressive kyphosis should be treated by anterior and posterior fusions.

Traumatic Spine Deformities

Trauma is a potent cause of deformity in the immature spine. It may be vertebral or extravertebral, accidental, non-accidental, or iatrogenic [1] (see Fig. 2.1) (see Chapters 5 and 6). The trauma of thoracoplasty or thoracotomy may cause spinal deformity, although it is nearly always very mild. Burns to the trunk, retroperitoneal fibrosis, or theco-peritoneal shunt syndrome can also cause deformity, the last usually a rather rigid hyperlordosis. It is, however, vertebral trauma that is most commonly associated with progressive deformity.

Deformities Caused by Infection

Infection in the immature spine is a potent cause of progressive kyphosis, with tuberculosis being much more serious than pyogenic infection (see Chapter 10 of General Principles of Children's Orthopaedic Disease). Most pyogenic infections produce a spontaneous interbody fusion with little in the way of spinal asymmetry but tuberculosis is quite different: there is much more disc and endplate destruction so that anterior spinal growth can be seriously impaired (Fig. 3.49). Thus, in the immature spine, progressive kyphosis is common, and, although anterior decompression and fusion may be required for the established disease or its neurological complications, anterior fusion itself produces further kyphosis.

Much has been learnt from the considerable experience of the tuberculous spine in Hong Kong [66]. The recommended treatment for tuberculous kyphosis is anterior discectomy above and below the kyphotic area with anterior strut and interbody grafting followed by second-stage segmental posterior stabilization.

Deformities Caused by Tumors

There are a number of ways in which tumors produce spinal deformities and in this respect intradural tumors, syringomyelia, extradural tumors, and the paravertebral tumors in childhood, plus the effect of their treatment, are all important considerations.

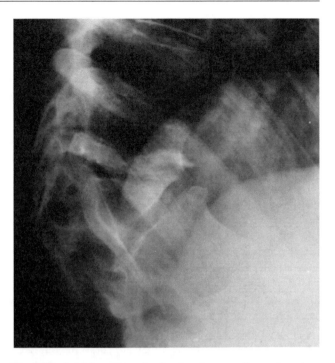

Fig. 3.49 Lateral radiograph showing long-standing tuberculous kyphosis since childhood. The owner is a distinguished orthopaedic surgeon!

Gliomas are the most common intradural neoplasm in children, followed by neuroblastomas and developmental hamartomas. Over half are benign and the cervical and thoracic spines are the sites of predilection. Back pain, limp, and leg weakness are common presenting symptoms and pathological reflexes, paralysis, and muscle spasm are common physical signs. Scoliosis is the presenting feature in 33% of cases. It is this combination of pain and scoliosis that should draw attention to the possibility of an underlying neoplasm (see Chapter 2).

Syringomyelia—pathological cavitation of the spinal cord—also commonly presents with a painful scoliosis, but headache is the most important associated symptom (see Fig. 2.12).

The spinal deformity which develops in association with intradural neoplasms and syringomyelia is of the idiopathic lordoscoliosis type and may be indistinguishable from true idiopathic scoliosis, although curve size and rotation are usually less obvious. Muscle spasm can make these deformities more rigid than would be expected. No particular side is favored and suspicion should be aroused by, for example, a progressive left thoracic deformity in a boy. With the more regular use of preoperative MRI scanning more and more syrinxes and cysts are being demonstrated although the pathological significance of some very small cysts is unknown. The message here is important: any painful or suspicious spinal deformity must be assessed by adequate imaging of the spinal canal contents (see Fig. 2.12).

Both syrinxes and intradural neoplasms require a posterior surgical approach by laminectomy which can produce a traumatic progressive kyphosis, particularly in the immature. Otherwise, decompression of the syrinx or excision of the tumor is generally accompanied by resolution of the idiopathic-type lordoscoliosis.

Extradural tumors such as aneurysmal bone cysts, giantcell tumors, and eosinophilic granulomas tend not to produce a spinal deformity, or only a very mild kyphosis. However, osteoblastoma or its smaller equivalent, the osteoid osteoma, is generally associated with a mild idiopathic-type lordoscoliosis, with the lesion sitting at the junction of the pedicle and transverse process on the concave side of the curve apex. Isotope bone scan typically show a "hot spot." Tomography or CT scanning defines the lesion precisely (see Chapter 5 General Principles of Children's Orthopaedic Disease) (see Fig. 2.13). Excision nearly always produces resolution of the deformity, although the posterior tethering effect of surgical scarring can sometimes induce further progression.

Wilms' tumor and neuroblastoma are the paravertebral tumors of childhood. Although they are paravertebral, radiation therapy can induce vertebral changes, particularly in the form of platyspondyly and a thoraco-lumbar kyphosis with a bullet-shaped vertebra. A true structural lordoscoliosis is, however, uncommon. Should progressive kyphosis require surgical treatment, previous spinal irradiation can increase the risk of pseudarthrosis after autogenous iliac crest grafting.

References

1. Leatherman KD, Dickson RA. Management of Spinal Deformities. Bristol: John Wright; 1988.
2. Adams W. Lectures on the Pathology and Treatment of Lateral and Other Forms of Curvature of the Spine. London: Churchill; 1865.
3. Dickson RA. Scoliosis: how big are you? Orthopaedics 1987; 10:881–887.
4. Cobb JR. Outline for the study of scoliosis. Am Acad Orthop Surg Instr Course Lect 1948; 5:261.
5. du Peloux J, Fauchet R, Faucon B, Stagnara P. Le plan d'election pour l'examen radiologique des cyphoscolioses. Rev Chirurg Orthop 1965; 51:517–524.
6. Goldstein LA, Waugh TR. Classification and terminology of scoliosis. Clin Orthop 1973; 93:10–22.
7. Branthwaite MA. Cardiorespiratory consequences of unfused idiopathic scoliosis. Br J Dis Chest 1986; 80:360–369.
8. Deacon P, Archer IA, Dickson RA. The anatomy of spinal deformity: a biomechanical analysis. Orthopaedics 1987; 10:897–903.
9. Dickson RA. Screening for scoliosis. Br Med J 1984; 289:269–270.
10. Somerville EW. Rotational lordosis: the development of the single curve. J Bone Joint Surg 1952; 34B:421–427.
11. Stirling J, Howel D, Millner PA, et al. Late-onset idiopathic scoliosis in children six to fourteen years old. J Bone Joint Surg 1996; 78A:1330–1336.
12. Sorenson KH. Scheuermann's juvenile kyphosis. Copenhagen: Munksgaard; 1964.
13. Archer IA, Dickson RA. Stature and idiopathic scoliosis. A prospective study. J Bone Joint Surg 1985; 67B:185–188.
14. Moe JH. A critical analysis of methods of fusion for scoliosis. J Bone Joint Surg 1958; 40A:529–554.
15. James JIP. Idiopathic scoliosis: the prognosis, diagnosis, and operative indications related to curve patterns and the age at onset. J Bone Joint Surg 1954; 36B:36–49.
16. Nachemson AL. A long term follow up study of non-treated scoliosis. Acta Orthop Scand 1968; 39:466–476.
17. Bengtsson G, Fallstrom K, Jansson B, Nachemson A. A psychological and psychiatric investigation of the adjustment of female scoliosis patients. Acta Psychiatrica Scand 1974; 50:50–59.
18. Whitby LG. Screening for disease. Definitions and criteria. Lancet 1974; ii:819–821.
19. Mardia KV, Walder AN, Berry E, et al. Assessing spinal shape. J Bone Joint Surg 1999; 61B:36–42.
20. Perdriolle R. La scoliose—son etude tridimensionnelle. Paris: Maloine; 1979.
21. Dickson RA. Spinal deformity—adolescent idiopathic scoliosis: nonoperative treatment. Spine 1999; 24:2601–2606.
22. Blount WP, Moe JH. The Milwaukee Brace. Baltimore: Williams & Wilkins; 1973.
23. Howell FR, Mahood J, Dickson RA. Growth beyond skeletal maturity. Spine 1992; 17:437–440.
24. Houghton GR, McInerney A, Tew A. Brace compliance in adolescent idiopathic scoliosis. J Bone Joint Surg 1987; 69B:852.
25. Miller JA, Nachemson AL, Schultz AB. Effectiveness of braces in mild idiopathic scoliosis. Spine J 1984; 5:362–373.
26. Watts HG, Hall JE, Stanish W. The Boston brace system for the treatment of low thoracic and lumbar scoliosis by the use of a girdle without superstructure. Clin Orthop 1977; 126:87–92.
27. Nachemson AL, Peterson L-E. Effectiveness of treatment with a brace in girls who have adolescent idiopathic scoliosis. J Bone Joint Surg 1995; 77A:815–822.
28. Peters L-E, Nachemson AL. Prediction of progression of the curve in girls who have adolescent idiopathic scoliosis of moderate severity. J Bone Joint Surg 1995; 77A:823–827.
29. Dickson RA, Weinstein SL. Bracing (and screening)—yes or no? Review Article. J Bone Joint Surg 1999; 81B:193–198.
30. Hibbs RA. An operation for progressive spinal deformities. NY Med J 1911; 93:1013–1016.
31. Harrington PR. Surgical instrumentation for management of scoliosis. J Bone Joint Surg 1960; 42A:1448.
32. American Orthopaedic Association Research Committee. End result study of the treatment of idiopathic scoliosis. J Bone Joint Surg 1941; 23:963–977.
33. Lenke LG, Betz RR, Harms J, et al. Adolescent idiopathic scoliosis: a new classification to determine extent of spinal arthrodesis. J Bone Joint Surg Am 2001; 83-A(8):1169–81.
34. Luque ER. The anatomic basis and development of segmental spinal instrumentation. Spine 1982; 7:256–259.
35. McMaster MJ, Macnicol MF. The management of progressive infantile idiopathic scoliosis. J Bone Joint Surg 1979; 61B:36–42.
36. Dubousset J, Graft H, Miladi L, Cotrel Y. Spinal and thoracic derotation with CD instrumentation. Orthop Trans 1986; 10:36.
37. Archer IA, Deacon P, Dickson RA. Idiopathic scoliosis in Leeds—a management philosophy. J Bone Joint Surg 1986; 68B:670.
38. Dwyer AF, Newton NC, Sherwood AA. An anterior approach to scoliosis: a preliminary report. Clin Orthop 1969; 62:192–202.
39. Griss P, Harms J, Zielke K. Ventral derotation spondylodesis (VDS). In: Dickson RA, Bradford DS, eds. Management of Spinal Deformities. London: Butterworths International Medical Reviews; 1984:193–236.
40. Dickson RA, Archer IA. Surgical treatment of late-onset idiopathic thoracic scoliosis. The Leeds procedure. J Bone Joint Surg 1987; 69B:709–714.

41. Harrenstein RJ. Die Skoliose bei Saueglingen und ihre Behandlung. Z Orthop Chir 1930; 52:1–40.
42. Scott JC, Morgan TH. The natural history and prognosis of infantile idiopathic scoliosis. J Bone Joint Surg 1955; 37B: 400–413.
43. Lloyd-Roberts GC, Pilcher MF. Structural idiopathic scoliosis in infancy. J Bone Joint Surg 1965; 47B:520–523.
44. Mau H. Does infantile scoliosis require treatment? J Bone Joint Surg 1968; 50B:881.
45. Wynne-Davies R. Infantile idiopathic scoliosis. J Bone Joint Surg [B] 1975; 57:138–141.
46. Mehta MH. The rib vertebra angle in the early diagnosis between resolving and progressive infantile scoliosis. J Bone Joint Surg 1972; 54B:230–243.
47. Mehta MH, Morel G. The non-operative treatment of infantile idiopathic scoliosis. In: Zorab PA, Siegler D, eds. Scoliosis. London: Proceedings of the Sixth Symposium Academic; 1979: 71–84.
48. Mehta MH. Growth as a corrective force in the early treatment of progressive infantile scoliosis. J Bone Joint Surg 2005; 87B: 1237–1247.
49. Moe JH. A critical analysis of methods of fusion for scoliosis. J Bone Joint surg 1958; 40A:529–554.
50. Roaf R. The treatment of progressive scoliosis by unilateral growth arrest. J Bone Joint Surg 1963; 45B:637–651.
51. Andrew TA, Piggott H. Growth arrest for progressive scoliosis. J Bone Joint Surg 1996; 67B:193–197.
52. Thompson GH, Akbarnia BA, Campbell RM Jr. Growing rod techniques in early-onset scoliosis. J Pediatr Orthop 2007; 27(3): 354–361.
53. Verbout AJ. The Development of the Vertebral Column. Berlin: Springer; 1985.
54. McMaster MJ, Ohtsuka K. The natural history of congenital scoliosis. A study of 251 patients. J Bone Joint Surg 1982; 64A:1128–1147.
55. Leatherman KD, Dickson RA. Two-stage corrective surgery for congenital deformities of the spine. J Bone Joint Surg 1979; 61B:324–328.
56. Shapiro F, Bresnan MJ. Orthopaedic management of childhood neuromuscular disease. Part II: Peripheral neuropathies, Friedreich's ataxia, and arthrogryposis multiplex congenital. J Bone Joint Surg 1982; 64A:949–953.
57. Lonstein JE, Akbarnia BA. Operative treatment of spinal deformities in patients with cerebral palsy or mental retardation. J Bone Joint Surg 1983; 63A:43–55.
58. Shapiro F, Bresnan MJ. Orthopaedic management of childhood neuromuscular disease. Part I: Spinal muscular atrophy. J Bone Joint Surg 1982; 64A:785–789.
59. Aprin H, Bowen JR, MacEwen GD, Hall JE. Spine fusion in patients with spinal muscular atrophy. J Bone Joint Surg 1982; 64A:1179–1187.
60. Weimann RL, Gibson DA, Moseley CF, Jones DC. Surgical stabilization of the spine in Duchenne muscular dystrophy. Spine 1983; 8:776–780.
61. Winter RB, Moe JH, Bradford DS, et al. Spine deformity in neurofibromatosis. A review of 102 patients. J Bone Joint Surg 1979; 61A:677–694.
62. Benson DR, Donaldson DH, Millar EA. The spine in osteogenesis imperfecta. J Bone Joint Surg 1978; 60A:925–929.
63. Robins PR, Moe JH, Winter RB. Scoliosis in Marfan's syndrome, its characteristics and results of treatment in 35 patients. J Bone Joint Surg 1975 57A:358–368.
64. Kopits SE, Perovic MN, McKusick V, Robinson RA. Congenital atlanto-axial dislocations in various forms of dwarfism. J Bone Joint Surg 1972; 54A:1349–1350.
65. Nelson MA. Orthopaedic aspects of the chondrodystrophies. The dwarf and his orthopaedic problems. Ann Royal Coll Surg England 1970; 47:185–210.
66. Hodgson AR. Correction of kyphotic spinal deformities. J Bone Joint Surg 1973; 55B:211–212.

Chapter 4

Spondylolisthesis

Robert A. Dickson

Introduction

Spondylolisthesis is the slipping forward of one vertebra and the spine above it upon the vertebra immediately below. When the condition first received orthopaedic attention in the latter half of the twentieth century, it was believed to be of congenital origin, but now it is recognized that several varieties exist, most being acquired.

The International Society for Study of the Lumbar Spine proposed a classification that is now generally accepted [1]. Five types are recognized :

- dysplastic
- isthmic
- degenerative
- traumatic
- pathological

Degenerative spondylolisthesis affects the over 50-year-old age group and is attributable to instability of arthritic posterior facet joints. It is much more common in women, particularly at the L4–L5 level, and because the back of the spine is not left behind, it can lead to spinal stenosis.

Traumatic spondylolisthesis refers to forward subluxation of one vertebra upon another as the result of a fracture in a region other than the pars interarticularis, such as the pedicle. Taillard questioned whether this should be called spondylolisthesis, rather than simple traumatic vertebral subluxation [2].

Pathological spondylolisthesis may complicate a number of underlying conditions such as tuberculosis, giant cell tumor, Paget's disease, rheumatoid disease, Albers-Schönberg disease, arthrogryposis, syphilis, and metastases.

R.A. Dickson (✉)
Academic Unit of Orthopaedic Surgery, Leeds General Infirmary, Leeds, UK

In childhood and adolescence only the dysplastic and isthmic varieties are encountered. Both forms are strongly familial, with almost one-third of first-degree relations having the same lesion [3].

Isthmic Spondylolisthesis

The isthmus or pars interarticularis is the posterolateral bony element between the upper and the lower articular processes. There are three subtypes of isthmic spondylolisthesis classified as

- lytic
- attenuation of the pars
- acute pars fracture

However, there is little convincing evidence that acute fractures of the pars ever occur, and attenuation and elongation of the pars is seen only with dysplastic spondylolisthesis [4]. Therefore, for practical purposes, "isthmic spondylolisthesis" and "lytic spondylolisthesis" are interchangeable terms.

The defect in the pars interarticularis is referred to as a spondylolysis and slippage in lytic spondylolisthesis is the consequence of this defect (Fig. 4.1; see also Figs. 1.8, 1.9, and 1.10). The development of this defect was originally believed to be congenital, but lyses have been shown to be fatigue or stress fractures in what has been shown biomechanically to be the weakest part of the neural arch [5]. Although lyses have been noted in children younger than 2 years, these lesions do not generally develop until after the age of 5 years, with an increasing prevalence rate from 1 to 2% at this young end of the age spectrum to a constant 6–7% in the adult population, except in Eskimos who have a prevalence rate in excess of 50% [6]. Slippage (spondylolisthesis) probably only occurs in 10–20% of lyses. These fatigue fractures are much more common in those who pursue a particularly active life. Among gymnasts lyses occur in

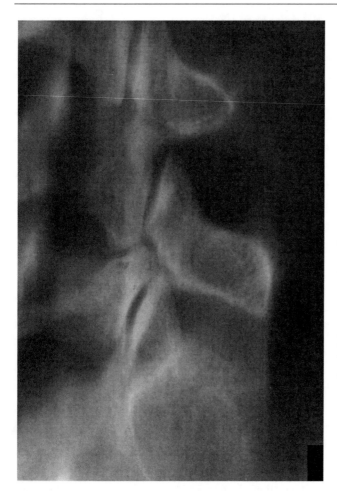

Fig. 4.1 Oblique lumbar tomogram showing a lysis in the pars interarticularis. The Scotty dog of LaChapelle has a collar

over 10% and spondylolisthesis in 6% [7]. Of course, these prevalence rates are derived from anteroposterior (AP) and lateral plain films of the spine and, if oblique tomograms or computed tomography (CT) were carried out, these rates would probably at least double. In contrast, the condition does not occur in those who, because of physical handicap, have never walked.

During childhood, the lytic region is filled with cartilage in which there are zones of endochondral ossification. Thus there is considerable potential for healing. Despite this, there is an increasing prevalence rate throughout growth. Once adulthood is reached, the nature of the spondylolysis changes toward that of a fracture non-union with hypertrophic callus (see Fig. 2.9), with little or no spontaneous healing potential. This explains the constant prevalence rate at maturity. In the adult, the appearance of the lytic defect should not therefore be misinterpreted as a gap, but rather as a mass lesion that may irritate the local nerve root. Radicular symptoms from lyses are not uncommon in the adult but are rare in the immature.

In the lumbar spine, forces are concentrated at the pars, particularly at the L5–S1 level, which is by far the most common site for spondylolisthesis [5].

Recently it has been shown that in the presence of a lysis the posterior facet joints are significantly more coronally orientated, thus producing a pincer-type effect, increasing forces across the pars [8] (Fig. 4.2).

Individuals with type II Scheuermann's disease (thoraco-lumbar kyphosis or apprentice's spine) have a much greater incidence of lower lumbar lyses, and these may be multiple.

When slippage occurs, the vertebral body in front of the lyses moves forward and leaves the back of the spinal arch behind. The spinal canal is therefore locally more capacious, quite unlike degenerative spondylolisthesis, and the step that is visible or palpable is at the junction of the slipped vertebra with the one above. Because the canal is large and the lyses cartilaginous, neurological symptoms and signs are very unusual.

As lytic spondylolisthesis is an acquired condition, both L5 and S1 are reasonably well formed and the slippage tends to be forward in the sagittal plane, without much in the way of local angular kyphosis (Fig. 4.3).

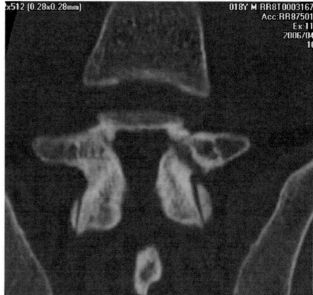

Fig. 4.2 Axial CT scan through the facet joints. On the side of the lysis the facet joint is more coronally orientated creating a pincer effect on movement

Dysplastic Spondylolisthesis

Originally termed "congenital," dysplastic spondylolisthesis is caused by hypoplasia or aplasia of the L5–S1 facet joints. The back of the spine is not left behind, so that the AP canal diameter is proportionately reduced. Interestingly, however,

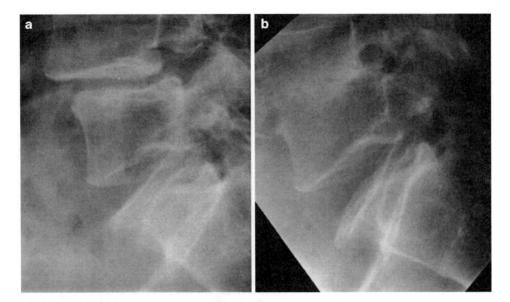

Fig. 4.3 (a) Lateral radiograph showing an L4/L5 lytic spondylolisthesis of long standing. These do not slip further after the attainment of maturity when they stabilize and produce no symptoms. (b) Over the course of the next year this man developed a septicemia and back pain. His L4/L5 discitis went on to spontaneous interbody fusion

only a modest degree of slippage occurs (usually not more than 25% of the sagittal width of the top of the sacrum) before a secondary spondylolysis develops in the pars of L5 which, although allowing further slippage to take place, does not further jeopardize the size of the spinal canal. Therefore, as with lytic spondylolisthesis, neurological symptoms and signs are unusual. It is only when secondary spondylolysis complicates dysplastic spondylolisthesis that attenuation of the pars can be seen before a frank spondylolysis develops [4] (Fig. 4.4).

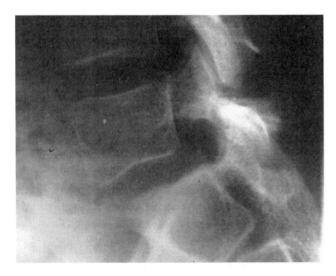

Fig. 4.4 Lateral radiograph of the lower lumbar spine with an L5/S1 dysplastic spondylolisthesis (note the lordotic-shaped L5 and the reciprocal rounding of the upper border of the sacrum anteriorly). The pars on each side have stretched and a secondary lysis has developed

Because the condition is congenital and develops at an earlier age than lytic spondylolisthesis, the body of L5 and the upper sacrum may be considerably deformed. The L5 vertebra becomes increasingly wedge shaped and the upper sacrum rounds off. Furthermore, in dysplastic spondylolisthesis there is always a spina bifida occulta of L5 or S1 and the sacrum appears more open than normal. It is these radiographic features on both AP and lateral projections that clearly differentiate the dysplastic from the lytic variety (Fig. 4.5). Because the L5 and S1 vertebrae are reciprocally misshapen, the slippage in dysplastic spondylolisthesis is very much more a progressive kyphosis than a simple slip forward in the sagittal plane.

Measurement

It has become the accepted standard to measure the degree of spondylolisthesis on a standing lateral radiograph [9]. Although a variety of measurements have been described, two are of particular value:

1. The extent of anterior displacement or slip.
2. The angle of sagittal rotation, also known as the sagittal roll, slip angle, or lumbo-sacral kyphosis (Fig. 4.6).

The extent of anterior displacement is the distance between the posterior cortex of L5 and the posterior cortex of S1, expressed as a percentage of the anteroposterior diameter of S1.

Fig. 4.5 AP radiograph of the lumbo-sacral junction in a severe dysplastic spondylolisthesis. Note the upside down appearance of Napoleon's hat as the sacrum overlaps L5. Observe the obligatory spina bifida occulta

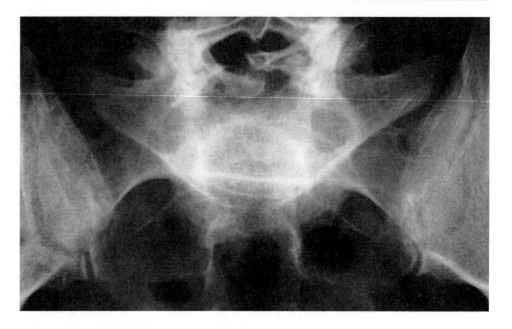

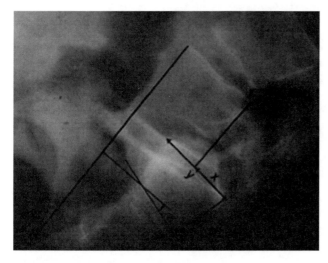

Fig. 4.6 Radiological measurement of spondylolisthesis. (i) Anterior displacement—the degree of slip forward of L5 is expressed as a percentage, $x/y \times 100$. (ii) Sacral inclination—angle a (the tilt of the sacrum from the vertical). (iii) Sagittal rotation—angle b (the angle subtended by L5 and S1 in the sagittal plane)

A more important clinical correlation is the angle of sagittal rotation, which is the relationship between L5 and S1 as subtended by lines drawn parallel to the anterior cortex of L5 and the posterior cortex of S1. The important clinical deformity in spondylolisthesis is lumbo-sacral kyphosis. The angle of sagittal rotation more accurately defines the clinical problem as a very considerable lytic spondylolisthesis with, say, a 75% slip purely in the sagittal plane may produce no clinical deformity whatever.

Clinical Features

Patients present with pain, deformity, neurological symptoms, hamstring tightness, and gait abnormality. The low back pain is mechanical, being worse during activity and hyperextension and relieved by rest. The pain is often referred to the buttock and thigh, but rarely with radicular distribution into the leg. Hamstring spasm or contracture is commonly associated with the more severe degrees of spondylolisthesis, particularly of the dysplastic variety, in which progressive lumbo-sacral kyphosis leads to relative flexion of the hip and knee; in severe degrees of slippage, there is frank hamstring contracture over and above any spasm induced by local discomfort. As the lumbo-sacral kyphosis progresses and the hips and knees take up a Z-deformity, posture becomes increasingly more distressing. Occasionally, with spondyloptosis, the L5 body finishes anterior to the first sacral segment, allowing the upper posterior corner of S1 to indent the canal, producing symptoms of spinal claudication and leg fatigue (Fig. 4.7). Otherwise, the only other neurological symptom encountered is occasional radicular pain in the same nerve root as the slipping vertebra (i.e., L5 for an L5–S1 slip and L4 for an L4–L5 slip).

Above the lumbo-sacral kyphosis, a compensatory thoraco-lumbar hyperlordosis may develop, with an anterior skin crease at umbilical level. Thus from the top of the spine down to the feet a gradually increasing Z-deformity can occur. Neurological examination is usually normal, but attention should be directed to the relevant nerve root. During adolescence, these children may suffer a spondylolisthetic

Fig. 4.7 (**a**) Lateral radiograph of the lumbo-sacral region showing a spondyloptosis with L5 lying in front of S1. (**b**) Sagittal MRI slice showing that, as usual, despite the severe deformity the spinal canal is capacious because secondary lyses have left the back of the spine behind. (**c**) Side view of this girl showing no significant deformity. (**d**) Front view showing the abdominal skin crease because severe dysplastic spondylolisthesis is effectively a kyphosis. (**e**) Forward bending view revealing the obvious kyphosis. She was in no pain and had normal function

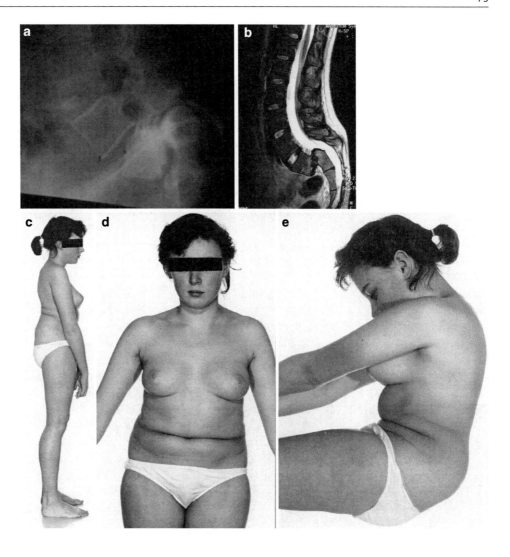

"crisis" [4], with profound muscle spasm such that patients can be deformed in the frontal plane in addition to their lateral profile. Lesions at the L4–L5 level tend to have a worse prognosis than those at the L5–S1 level, in terms of both irritability and progression.

Treatment

As with most orthopaedic conditions, there is a considerable divergence of opinion as to how patients should be treated. Recent years have seen an exponential increase in the use of operative surgery, particularly in the nature of attempted reduction with transpedicular instrumentation in addition to biological fusion. In many countries, such techniques are currently accepted as standard, but there is no convincing evidence that patients fare better.

There is a place for both conservative and operative management. For the immature patient with a spondylolysis and considerable potential for healing, an expectant policy should

be pursued. The child presenting with mechanical low back pain whose plain radiographs indicate no obvious abnormality and in whom there is no suspicion of any underlying bone destructive lesion (e.g., absence of night pain) should have oblique films taken of the lumbar spine. If necessary, CT scanning with the gantry angle appropriate for the pars (see Fig. 2.9) rather than the intervertebral disc is useful for demonstrating spondylolyses. Spondylolyses with active cartilaginous endochondral ossification zones can be detected with isotope bone scanning.

Many patients with mechanical low back pain do not have a satisfactory diagnosis even after exhaustive investigation, and it is important to bear in mind the possibility of a spondylolysis. As patients approach maturity, they are also vulnerable to intervertebral disc derangements and the two frequently coexist. Therefore in the older adolescent it is important to take a careful history, with particular reference to nerve root compression. Exuberant tissue around the spondylolysis may compress the local nerve root (L5 for the L5–S1 level) (see Fig. 2.9), the same root that will be affected by an L4–L5 disc prolapse. It is therefore quite wrong to rush in to surgical treatment at the level of the spondylolisthesis without careful imaging of the adjacent motion segments.

As the majority of spondylolyses heal, or at least become asymptomatic with the passage of time, the condition should be treated symptomatically. Many patients are sporting individuals and a period of rest which, if unsuccessful, can be followed by injecting the lysis with painkiller and anti-inflammatory drugs can often be successful. For particularly recalcitrant cases the lyses can be fused with screws or compression hooks (Fig. 4.8). Wiltse has a very considerable experience of spondylolysis and spondylolisthesis and advises that treatment of a spondylolysis or a spondylolisthesis of less than 25% should be confined to a period of rest for the acute exacerbation [10]. If the degree of slip is less than 50%, sporting activities are not restricted. A concern to many is the risk of further slippage if surgical treatment is not carried out, but long-term studies have shown that progressive slippage occurs only during the first few years [10]. If the degree of slippage is 30% or less at presentation, then further slipping is unusual.

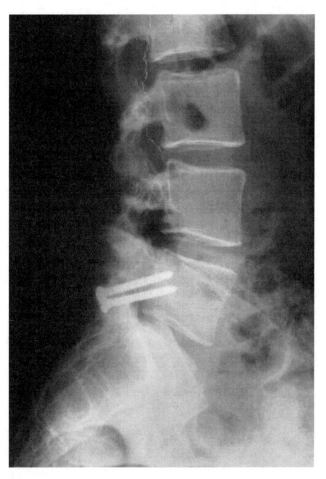

Fig. 4.8 Lateral radiograph of the lumbar spine showing a Buck's fusion for bilateral lyses

If a child has a slip of more than 50% or intractable local symptoms, spinal fusion is indicated (Fig. 4.9). Wiltse and Jackson advise bilateral intertransverse fusion in situ without instrumentation and have reported excellent results in 90% of cases [10]. Bilateral intertransverse fusion is preferred to either anterior or posterior fusion, for both biomechanical and clinical reasons [11]. The fusion rate is greater and further slippage after surgery is unusual. For those with neurological symptoms, nerve root decompression and removal of the loose, "rattle" fragment can be performed, but Wiltse and Jackson state that these symptoms always resolve with a solid fusion [10]. Interbody fusion should be reserved for the occasional patient in whom bilateral intertransverse fusion has failed; although usually performed anteriorly, this procedure can also be performed posteriorly [12].

Wiltse and Jackson also demonstrated clearly that lumbar and hamstring muscle spasm resolves with solid fusion, and body shape improves without the need for reduction [10] (Fig. 4.9). The more severe the slip, and the more severe the clinical disability, the more tempting is the desire to correct the condition surgically. However, with lytic spondylolisthesis the deformity is seldom significant, and what muscle spasm exists in the erector spinae or hamstrings settles with a sound fusion. As lumbo-sacral kyphosis is more important than percentage slip, reduction is particularly attractive in significant dysplastic spondylolisthesis. In 1932, Capener first attempted open reduction of a spondylolisthesis [13], and since then various open and closed techniques have been advanced. In 1969, Harrington used his scoliosis instrumentation in an effort to reduce spondylolisthesis and designed and implanted transpedicular screws attached to his rods in an unsuccessful attempt to correct the position of the displaced vertebrae [14]. Segmental wiring techniques became popular and were followed by staged anterior and posterior multiple procedures, some of which corrected the slippage at the expense of the L5 nerve root [15].

It would seem logical to try closed reduction first and, if that fails and reduction is still considered important, to proceed to operative reduction. The Scaglietti closed cast system can be very effective, although it is time-consuming for the patient [16]. A localizer cast similar to that used for scoliosis is applied under traction on a Risser–Cotrel table, with the spine extended at the lumbo-sacral region as much as can be tolerated. The addition of a spica round one thigh maintains the spine–pelvis relationship. Lateral radiographs taken before and after casting demonstrate whether a reduction is being achieved. Further casts are applied over the ensuing weeks until no further correction is obtained. Bilateral intertransverse fusion is then performed in the cast, which is retained until the fusion consolidates.

Should this technique be unsuccessful, operative reduction can be achieved, but it is necessary to visualize clearly

Fig. 4.9 (**a**) Lateral radiograph of the lumbo-sacral region showing a dysplastic spondylolisthesis on the point of going in front of the sacrum. (**b**) Side view of this 15-year-old boy. He had severe pain and spasm with no back movements at all. This is called the adolescent crisis.
(**c**) PA radiograph of the lumbar spine showing a scoliosis secondary to muscle spasm. (**d**) Lateral radiograph taken a year after Scaglietti cast treatment showing a good correction and a sound posterior fusion.
(**e**) PA radiograph 1 year after surgery. All pain and spasm had been completely relieved. Note the sound ala-transverse fusion. There is no need for metalwork

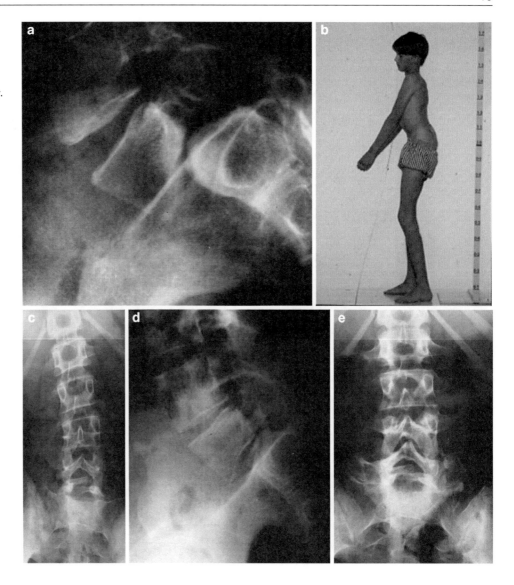

the L5 nerve roots during the procedure. In fact, the instability produced locally by thorough visualization of the L5 roots from cauda equina to foramen allows a degree of reduction to occur spontaneously on the operating table.

The end point of surgical treatment for spondylolisthesis has to be a sound spinal fusion, and the addition of rigid internal fixation may enhance the fusion rate. While there are distinct advantages in rigidly fixing the spine internally, from the point of view of earlier mobility without a cumbersome cast, it has to be asked whether, if a Wiltse-type fusion in situ without metalwork allows successful fusion in over 90%, can the addition of metalwork be regarded as either justified or advantageous?

References

1. Wiltse LL, Newman PH, Macnab I. Classification of spondylolysis and spondylolisthesis. Clin Orthop Rel Res 1976; 117:23–29.
2. Taillard WF. Etiology of spondylolisthesis. Clin Orthop Rel Res 1978; 117:30–39.
3. Wynne-Davies R, Scott JHS. Inheritance and spondylolisthesis. A radiographic family survey. J Bone Joint Surg 1979; 61B:301–305.
4. Scott JHS. Spondylolisthesis. In: Dickson RA, ed. Spinal Surgery: Science and Practice. London: Butterworths; 1990:353–367.
5. Shah JS, Hampson WGJ, Jayson MIV. The distribution of surface strain in the cadaveric lumbar spine. J Bone Joint Surg 1978; 60B:246–251.
6. Stewart TD. The age incidence of neural arch defects in Alaskan natives, considered from the standpoint of etiology. J Bone Joint Surg 1953; 35A:937–950.
7. Jackson DW, Wiltse LL, Cirincione RJ. Spondylolysis in the female gymnast. Clin Orthop 1976; 117:68–73.
8. Rankine JJ, Dickson RA. An investigation of the facet joint anatomy in spondylolysis. Musculoskeletal Scientific Session 1.

Proceedings of the UK Radiology Congress 2008. British Institute of Radiology.

9. Wiltse LL , Winter RB. Terminology and measurement of spondylolisthesis. J Bone Joint Surg 1983; 65A:768–772.

10. Wiltse LL, Jackson DW. Treatment of spondylolisthesis and spondylolysis in children. Clin Orthop Rel Res 1976; 117:92–100.

11. Lee CK, Langrana NA. Lumbosacral spinal fusion. A biomechanical study. Spine 1984; 9:574–581.

12. Cloward RB. Lesions of the intervertebral disks and their treatment by interbody fusion methods. Clin Orthop Rel Res 1963; 27:51–77.

13. Capener N. Spondylolisthesis. B J Surg 1932; 19:374–386.

14. Harrington PR, Tullos. Spondylolisthesis in children. Observations and surgical treatment. Clin Orthop Rel Res HS 1971; 79:75–84.

15. Bradford DS. Treatment of severe spondylolisthesis. A combined approach for reduction and stabilisation. Spine 1979; 4:423–429.

16. Scaglietti O, Frontino C, Bartolozzi P. Technique of anatomical reduction of lumbar spondylolisthesis and its surgical stabilisation. Clin Orthop Rel Res 1976; 117:164–175.

Chapter 5

Traumatic Disorders of the Cervical Spine

Robert N. Hensinger

Introduction

The child's cervical spine often presents a diagnostic dilemma. The presence of cervical growth plates, lack of complete ossification, unique developmental aspects, and hypermobility are causes of confusion in the interpretation of cervical radiographs in children with neck pain or stiffness [1]. Cervical spine radiographs in children are notoriously difficult to interpret. Lack of familiarity with normal growth and development and poorly positioned films make diagnosis difficult and can lead to problems in management [2].

Normal Development and Variations

Knowledge of normal physeal development is essential when interpreting a child's radiograph. Physeal plates are generally smooth, regular, in predicted locations, and have subchondral sclerotic lines. Fractures are irregular, without sclerosis, and usually in unpredictable locations. The upper two cervical vertebrae are unique in their development (Fig. 5.1); the remaining five develop essentially uniformly.

Upper Cervical Vertebrae (C1 and C2)

At birth the atlas is composed of three ossification centers—one for the body (anterior ring) and one for each of the two neural arches. The anterior ring is occasionally bifid and is not usually present at birth, appearing during the first year of life (Fig. 5.1). On rare occasions it is absent and may

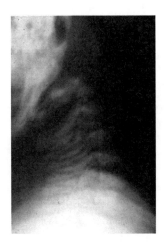

Fig. 5.1 An extension radiograph of a 6-week-old child; the anterior arch of the atlas may slide upward to protrude beyond the ossified part of the dens, giving a mistaken impression of odontoid hypoplasia. Note that the anterior portion of the ring of C1 is not yet ossified

close by fusion of the neural arches anteriorly. The posterior arch of the first cervical vertebra usually closes by the third year. Occasionally its development is incomplete or remains completely absent throughout life. The neurocentral synchondroses link the neural arches to the body of the atlas and are best seen in the open-mouth view. They close by the seventh year of life and should not be mistaken for fractures [2].

The developing axis has four ossification centers at birth; one for each neural arch, one (occasionally two) for the body, and another for the dens. In the anteroposterior (AP) open-mouth view of a young child, the dens (odontoid process) is "sandwiched" between the neural arches. It surmounts the body of the axis and is separated from it by a synchondrosis, or vestigial disc space of the odontoid. Below this are the synchondroses between the body and the neural arches, which together combine to form the letter H.

The epiphysis or synchondrosis of the odontoid runs well below the level of the articular processes of the axis. In the adult, a persistent epiphyseal line is not seen at the base of the odontoid process where fractures often occur, but within the

R.N. Hensinger (✉)
Department of Orthopaedic Surgery, University of Michigan, Ann Arbor, MI, USA

body of the axis well below the level of the articular facets. Cattell and Filtzer [1] found that this basilar epiphysis of the odontoid may persist up to 11 years of age as a narrow, sclerotic line and can resemble an undisplaced fracture.

The odontoid fuses with the neural arches and the body of the axis between 3 and 6 years of age, essentially the same time that the remainder of the vertebral body joins the neural arches. Therefore, no epiphysis or synchondrosis should be present in the axis in the open-mouth view of a child over 6 years of age. The normal synchondrosis between the dens and the arch of C2 is not seen on the lateral view of the cervical spine, but is easily visible on the oblique view and should not be mistaken for a fracture [3]. The ossification center of the inferior vertebral ring (ring apophysis) of the second cervical vertebra should cause little confusion. It ossifies during the late years of childhood and fuses with the body at approximately 25 years of age.

The tip of the odontoid is not ossified at birth and it has a V-shaped appearance. A mistaken impression of odontoid hypoplasia may be given by a lateral extension radiograph in a very young child because the anterior arch of the atlas slides upward and protrudes beyond the ossified portion of the dens to lie against the unossified tip [1] (Fig. 5.1). A small ossification center, known as the summit ossification center, appears at its tip at age 3–6 years and fuses with the main portion or the odontoid by age 12 years. Its persistence is referred to as an ossiculum terminale and should not be confused with an os odontoideum [4].

Lower Cervical Vertebrae (C3–C7)

The third to seventh cervical vertebrae ossify from three centers: one from the body and one from each neural arch. The neural arches close at the second or third year, and the neurocentral synchondroses between the neural arches and the vertebral body fuse from the third to sixth years. In the lateral radiograph, the ossified portion of the vertebral body in the young child is wedge-shaped until it becomes squared off at about 7 years of age [1]. The bodies, neural arches, and pedicles enlarge radially by periosteal apposition, similar to the periosteal growth seen in long bones.

At birth, the vertebral bodies possess superior and inferior cartilage plates firmly bonded to the disc [5]. The interface between vertebral body and endplate is similar to the physis of a long hone. The vertebral body is analogous to the metaphysis and the clear space between it and the endplate represents the physeal plate where longitudinal growth occurs [6]. Clinically as well as experimentally, stress applied to the vertebral bodies results in splitting of the cartilage endplate at the growth zone in the area of columnar

and calcified cartilage rather than at the stronger junction between it and the vertebral disc.

The apophyseal rings on the upper and lower surfaces of the vertebral body begin to ossify late in childhood and fuse to the vertebral body by the age of 25 years. Apophyseal fractures in the cervical spine have been reported. The inferior endplates are believed to be more susceptible to fracture than the superior because of the mechanical protection afforded by the developing uncinate processes [7].

Mobility

The cervical region is normally the most flexible area of the spine, especially in children. It may be difficult to determine normal from abnormal mobility in a young child's neck. The most mobile articulation in the cervical spine is between the atlas and axis. Half of all cervical rotation occurs here. Some side-to-side bending is also present, but hyperextension is limited by the dens. In 3- to 10-year-old children, subluxation is present if there is more than 10° of forward flexion at C1–C2 or if the distance between the posterior spines or C1 and C2 is greater than 10 mm in the neutral radiograph. The atlanto-occipital joint allows some flexion and extension but very little rotation. The C2–C3 joint is slightly mobile in flexion and extension, but not in rotation. Thus, the relatively mobile C1–C2 joint is located between two relatively stiff joints. This concentrates forces at the atlanto-axial joint, and partly explains the high percentage of cervical injuries at this level.

The anterior arch of the atlas is firmly held against the odontoid process by the transverse atlantal ligament [8]. This space is called the atlanto-dens interval (ADI) and on the lateral radiograph is measured from the anterior edge of the dens to the posterior edge of the anterior arch of the atlas (Fig. 5.2). Further stability is provided by accessory ligaments such as the alar ligaments that connect the tip of the odontoid process with the medial aspect of the occipital condyles and the capsular ligaments. In the adult, anterior displacement of the ring of C1 up to 3 mm from the odontoid is within the range of normal [8]. When the distance between the odontoid process and the anterior arch of C1 is 4.5 mm or greater, the transverse ligament is ruptured and when the distance is 10–12 mm, all ligaments have failed [8]. Radiographic surveys of children suggest that an ADI of up to 4 mm may be normal [9]. (If the space between the dens and anterior arch of C1 is not symmetrical on the flexion view, the ADI should he measured at the mid-portion of the dens.) The larger normal limit in children is probably due to greater ligamentous laxity and incomplete ossification. A slight increase in the neutral ADI may indicate an injury of

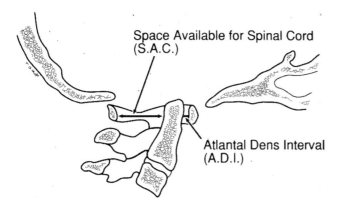

Fig. 5.2 Sagittal views of the atlanto-axial joint demonstrating the atlanto-dens interval (ADI). The space available for the cord (SAC) is the distance between the posterior aspect of the odontoid and the posterior ring of C1. From: Hensinger RN, Fielding JW. The cervical spine. In: Morrisey RT (ed). Lovell and Winter's Pediatric Orthopaedics, 3rd edition, 1990:718

the transverse atlantal ligament. This can be a useful sign of acute injury, where flexion-extension views are potentially hazardous.

The ADI is not helpful in chronic atlanto-axial instability due to congenital anomalies, rheumatoid arthritis, or Down's syndrome. In these conditions, the odontoid is frequently found to be hypermobile with a widened ADI, particularly in flexion [10] (Fig. 5.3). Here attention should be directed to the amount of space available for the spinal cord (SAC) by measuring the distance from the posterior aspect of the odontoid or axis to the nearest posterior structure (foramen magnum or posterior ring of the atlas) (Fig. 5.2).

This measurement is particularly helpful in non-union of the odontoid or os odontoideum because the ADI may be normal in either condition, yet in flexion or extension there is considerable reduction in the space available for the spinal cord (Fig. 5.4). McRae [11] measured the distance from the posterior aspect of the odontoid to either the posterior arch of the atlas or the posterior lip of the foramen magnum, whichever was closer (Fig. 5.2). He found that a neurological deficit was present if this distance was less than 19 mm. It should be measured in flexion because this position most dramatically reduces the SAC.

Patients with a normal odontoid process and an attenuated or ruptured transverse atlantal ligament are particularly at risk; with anterior shift of the atlas over the axis, the spinal cord is easily damaged by direct impingement against the intact odontoid process.

Steel [12] called attention to the check-rein effect of the alar ligaments and how they form the second line of defense after disruption of the transverse atlantal ligament. This secondary stability no doubt plays an important role in patients with chronic atlanto-axial instability. Steel defined the *rule of thirds;* he recognized that the area of the vertebral canal at the first cervical vertebra can be divided into one-third cord, one-third odontoid, and one-third "space" [12]. The one-third spinal space represents a safe zone in which displacement can occur without neurological impingement and is roughly equivalent to the transverse diameter of the odontoid [4]. In chronic atlanto-axial instability it is important to recognize when the patient has exceeded the "safe zone" and enters the area of impending spinal cord compression. At this point the second line of defense, the alar ligaments, has failed and there is no longer a margin of safety.

Fig. 5.3 Atlanto-axial instability with intact odontoid. (**a**) Extension—the ADI and SAC return to normal as the intact odontoid provides a bony block to subluxation in hyperextension. From: Hensinger RN, Fielding JW. The cervical spine. In: Morrisey RT (ed). Lovell and Winter's Pediatric Orthopaedics, 3rd edition, 1990:718. (**b**) Flexion—forward sliding of the atlas with an increased ADI and decreased SAC

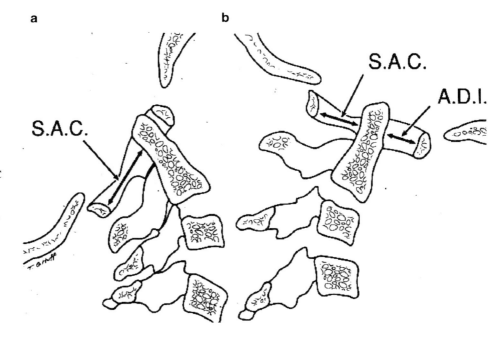

Fig. 5.4 Atlanto-axial
instability with os odontoideum,
absent odontoid, or traumatic
non-union. (**a**) Extension—
posterior subluxation with
reduction in SAC and no change
in the ADI. From: Hensinger RN,
Fielding JW. The cervical spine.
In: Morrisey RT (ed). Lovell and
Winter's Pediatric Orthopaedics,
3rd edition, 1990:719. (**b**)
Flexion—forward sliding of the
atlas with reduction of the SAC,
but no change in ADI

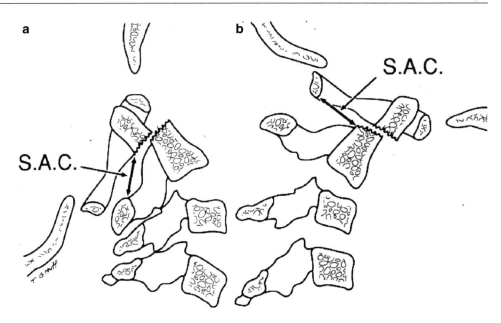

Pseudosubluxation

One of the most frequently misinterpreted findings on paediatric cervical spine films is hypermobility of C2 on C3
in flexion. While this injury pattern can occur in children,
the more common explanation is C2–C3 pseudosubluxation
(Fig. 5.5). Cattell and Filtzer [1] reported that 9% of children between the ages of 1 and 16 years (19% of children
from 1 to 7 years) had marked forward displacement of
C2 on C3 in flexion, "clearly resembling" a subluxation.
Forty percent of normal children under the age of 8 years
demonstrated a definite tendency toward excessive anterior
displacement of C2 on C3 in flexion. While pseudosubluxation is a well-recognized phenomenon in small children, it
has also been reported in teenagers.

Swischuck [13] described the importance of the posterior
cervical (spinolaminar) line (Fig. 5.5) as a helpful guide
to differentiate pathological subluxation from normal pseudosubluxation. The posterior cervical line in flexion and
extension should have all three of the anterior edges or the
spinous processes of C1, C2, and C3 line up within 1 mm of
each other [9].

The facet joint angles are shallow in children. This relative
flatness adds to the greater mobility and forward transla-
tional motion that children demonstrate in their cervical spine
(Fig. 5.5).

Lower Cervical Instability

The criteria for lower cervical instability in the adult have
been delineated by White et al. [14] in their classic study in
1975, but may not be entirely appropriate for the young child.

In children, the interspinous distance posteriorly can help
to diagnose traumatic ligamentous tears. At any given level,
the interspinous distance may be 1.5 times greater than the
distance one level above or below [9]. Increased interspinous
distance, divergence of the articular processes, and widening of the posterior aspect of the disc space are indicative of
instability in paediatric cervical spine injuries [9].

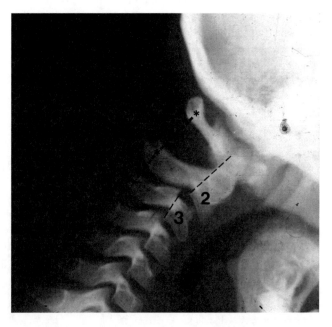

Fig. 5.5 Pseudosubluxation of C2 on C3. Hypermobility is common
in children under the age of 8 years. Specific measurement of the movement of the vertebral bodies (*thin dotted line*) is unreliable whereas the
relationship with the posterior elements (*thick dotted line*) is more consistent. [13] In flexion the posterior arch of C2 lies in a relatively straight
line with C1 and C3. Note the relative horizontal nature of the facet
joints which allows greater mobility

Retropharyngeal Soft Tissues

The space between the cervical spine and the pharynx in the region of C3 has been estimated to be a maximum of 5 mm in adults. An increase in width after trauma is presumptive evidence of hemorrhage or edema secondary to fracture or dislocation. Wholey and associates [15] suggest 3.5 mm for the normal retropharyngeal space (opposite the inferior base of C6) as the average value for normal children under 15 years. They suggest further investigation if the retropharyngeal space is wider than 7 mm and the retrotracheal space is over 22 mm.

In inspiration the pharyngeal wall is close to the vertebra while in forced expiration there may be a marked "physiological" increase in the width of the retropharyngeal soft tissue shadow. Crying displaces the hyoid bone and the larynx forward and will increase the width of this shadow.

Cervical Spine Injuries

General Principles

The cervical spine in the adolescent responds to trauma in the same way as in adults. In general, children under the age of 8 years have a higher incidence of injury to the upper cervical spine than the adolescent or adult [16]. The synchondroses tend to be involved. Facet fractures or vertebral dislocations are rare. By the age of 8–10 years the bony cervical spine has approached adult configuration and most of the cartilage lines have disappeared with the exception of the vertebral ring apophyses. The emphasis, in this section, is on the child's spine from birth to age 10 years.

Incidence and Physical Findings

Injuries to the child's cervical spine are rare and most commonly found in the upper cervical region above C3. Hause et al. [17] reviewed 228 patients with cervical spine or spinal cord injury and found only 10 children under the age of 15 with 70% of children's lesions in the atlas and axis compared with 16% in adults. A more recent review revealed similar findings, with 68% of the injuries in C1–C4 and 25% in C5–C7 [18].

In most series of paediatric cervical fractures, there is a relatively low incidence of neurological deficit, and neurological involvement has a better prognosis in children compared to adults [19]. The younger children tend to sustain more neurological injuries than older teenage patients [20].

In young children, falls and motor vehicle accidents (52%) are the predominant etiology [18, 21]. In older children, sports-related injuries (27%) become more frequent, with football accounting for 29% of all these injuries [18]. Eleraky et al. [19] reported that neck injuries are often associated with trauma to other portions of the body, particularly the head and face (40%) [21, 22]. Evidence of head or facial trauma, especially in the comatose patient, should alert the physician to hidden cervical spine injury (Fig. 5.6). Furnival et al. [23]

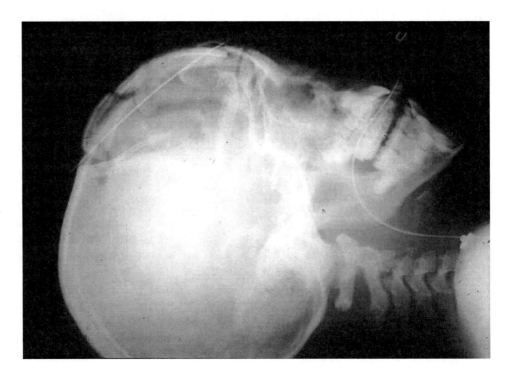

Fig. 5.6 Supine lateral radiograph of a 6-year-old child struck by an automobile. There is an unstable teardrop fracture of the body of C3, with kyphosis at the fracture site (C3). Cervical injuries in children are often associated with head or facial trauma as seen in this case of a massive depressed skull fracture. From: Herzenberg JE, Hensinger RN. Pediatric cervical spine injuries. Trauma Quarterly 1989; 5:73–81. Used with permission

reported a high incidence of neck injuries with the use of trampolines. Gonzalez et al. [24] noted that clinical examination of the neck may help to determine significant cervical spine injury in the awake and alert blunt trauma patient. Somatosensory evoked potentials (SSEPs) can be helpful in detecting a spinal cord injury, especially in children with head injuries and in a comatose patient [16].

Radiological Evaluation

Rachesky et al. [25] attempted to identify which injured children require cervical radiographs by reviewing a large series (2133), in which 25 (1.2%) had a documented cervical spine injury They concluded that cervical spine radiographs were indicated if the child had complained of neck pain or if there was head or facial trauma associated with a motor vehicle accident (Fig. 5.6). Whenever the diagnosis of a localized cervical spine injury is made, a careful examination should be made of the remaining cervical spine, as in children there is a high incidence (24%) of multiple level injury (Fig. 5.7). Avellino et al. [2] reported on the misdiagnosis of synchondroses and cervical spine injuries in children over a 12-year period and found that 19% of these injuries were misdiagnosed; 5% were missed fractures and 14% were normal or developmental variations interpreted to be fractures or dislocations. The error rate for infants and children under 8 years of age was 24%, while for children over 9 years of age the error rate was 15%. The occiput to C2 region was the most common site of diagnostic error, including the hangman's fracture or missed C1 ring fracture of the spine.

Further imaging, particularly flexion-extension lateral radiographs, may be required to assess stability. Tomograms

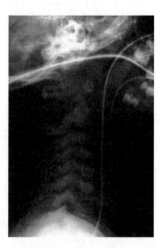

Fig. 5.7 Cervical injury in a 3-year-old. Initial lateral radiograph in traction demonstrating multiple injuries of the cervical spine. Note the distraction at occiput-C1, C1–C2, and C6–C7

have been used to assess the extent of the bony injury, but have been largely replaced by computed tomography (CT). In the past, CT was not recommended as a screening tool [26]. Sanchez et al. [27] recommend using helical CT scans and eliminating plain radiographs. Selective use of CT scanning increased the accuracy of detecting cervical spine injuries from 54 to 100%.

CT may identify occult fractures in the posterior elements that are not clearly seen or appreciated on radiographs. As there is such a high incidence of cervical spine injuries in patients with severe, blunt multiple injury, CT scan can be helpful particularly in the intensive care unit. Woodring noted that, while CT scans were particularly helpful for C1–C2 problems, plain films were better at detecting fractures of the vertebral body, dens, and spinous processes, and subluxation and dislocation [28]. However, plain films may show a vertebral body fracture where CT would show an additional fracture through the posterior elements of the same vertebra. CT is recommended for all fractures of C1 and C7-T1 when plain films are not helpful [29] and for surgical planning. If the patient has a normal CT scan, but a neurological deficit is present, then magnetic resonance imaging (MRI) should be used [27].

CT scans, particularly with flexion and extension views, are very useful to demonstrate atlanto-occipital dislocation, subluxation of the vertebral bodies, and fractures of the lateral masses and processes.

Spinal Cord Injury Without Observable Radiographic Abnormalities

It is well recognized that children may have partial or complete paralysis without radiographic evidence of spine fracture or dislocation. Pang and Wilberger [30] coined the phrase "spinal cord injury without observable radiographic abnormalities" (SCIWORA). Yngve et al.[31] reported SCIWORA in 16 of 17 spinal cord injured children and noted that they tended to be younger than those with osseous fracture. Young children with SCIWORA typically have more severe neurological injury than older children [30–32].

MRI demonstrates parenchymal spinal cord injuries (Fig. 5.8) and disc herniation better than CT. Katzberg et al. [33] noted that MRI is more accurate than radiography in the detection of a wide spectrum of neck injuries [34]. It is superior for hemorrhage, edema, anterior/posterior longitudinal ligament injury, traumatic disc herniation, cord edema, and cord compression. CT remains preferable for the classification of bony injuries. In one study, the predominant neurological presentation of SCIWORA was a mild neurological deficit that resolved within 72 h [35]. MRI revealed

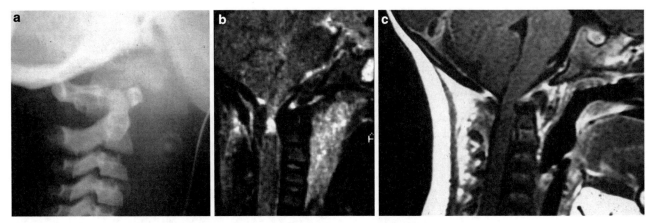

Fig. 5.8 (**a** and **b**) A 9-year-old who sustained an occiput-C1 dislocation in a motor vehicle accident. (**a**) Lateral radiograph demonstrating vertical displacement between the occiput and the ring of C1. (**b**) MRI of the same patient demonstrating a complete spinal cord injury at the level of occiput-C1. (**c**) CT scan of a 2-year-old male who was involved in a motor vehicle accident and sustained a fracture of the odontoid and a C1–C2 dislocation, which resulted in complete quadriplegia

abnormal features only in those patients with complete neurological deficits. These findings suggest that in the acute setting conventional MR images may lack the sensitivity to demonstrate neural and extraneural abnormalities associated with partial or temporary neurological deficits of SCIWORA even when those deficits persist beyond 72 h. MRI helps to exclude lesions that may require emergency decompression, such as hematomas and disc herniations and it serves as a prognosticator for neurological recovery [35]. Some children do not have paralysis immediately after trauma, but only after a latent period of 30 min to 4 days, apparently in the absence of further trauma. In Pang's study [16], the recurrent injury occurred mostly during the first 2 weeks after the initial SCIWORA, but one child had her recurrent injury at 10 weeks. In one large series, most patients' neurological status stabilized, but those who did develop a recurrence recovered back to a baseline [20]. The mean age of the SCIWORA diagnosis was 10.7 ± 4.6 years. Those who had recurrent SCIWORA were older, injured by low energy mechanisms, never had a positive MRI finding and had minor transient neurological deficits on both the initial and recurrent injuries. Twenty of 21 patients with recurrent SCIWORA were over the age of 8 years at the time of recurrence.

Every case of serious permanent SCIWORA had positive findings on CT or MRI [20] and it is very important to rule out spinal instability.

Neonatal Trauma

The normal infant is unable to support the head adequately until about 3 months of age. Infants, therefore, are incapable of protecting the cervical spine and spinal cord against excessive torsional and traction forces that may occur during delivery and the months following birth. Bony injury usually involves the upper cervical spine, but lower cervical injuries have been reported. These forces may exceed the stretch capability of the neck. According to Stern and Rand [36], the lax ligaments of a child's neck may not be able to protect the less elastic spinal cord, possibly explaining the occurrence of severe cord injuries without skeletal injury. Spinal cords removed from newborns dying from obstetric trauma show changes over long segments, suggesting that longitudinal traction was a major factor.

Skeletal injury due to obstetric trauma is probably underreported because the infantile spine, with its large percentage of cartilage, is difficult to evaluate radiologically, especially if the lesion occurs through cartilage or at the cartilage–bone interface. These injuries commonly occur in the absence of bony injury. They are usually associated (25%) with hyperextension of the fetal head in utero and during delivery [37]. Ultrasound and MRI can be helpful diagnostic tools. Early recognition of hyperextension of the fetal head in utero and a planned cesarean section are important preventive methods. If routine radiographs are normal, then flexion-extension views are necessary. MRI is better than CT in the diagnosis of upper cervical spinal cord compression. A cervical spine lesion should be considered in the differential diagnosis of infants who are found to be floppy at birth, particularly if the delivery was a difficult one. Complete flaccid paralysis with arreflexia is usually followed by the typical pattern of hyper-reflexia once spinal cord shock is over. Brachial plexus birth palsies also warrant a cervical spine radiograph.

Caffey [6] and Swischuck [38] described a form of child abuse called the "whiplash shaken infant syndrome." The weak infantile neck musculature cannot support the head when it is subjected to whiplash stresses. Intracranial and intraocular hemorrhages resulting in death, or latent cerebral injury, retardation, and permanent visual or hearing defects have been reported, together with fractures of the spine and spinal cord injuries.

Fig. 5.9 A 4-year-old who sustained a skull fracture and associated Jefferson fracture in a motor vehicle accident. CT of C1 shows the ring broken at two sites (FX)

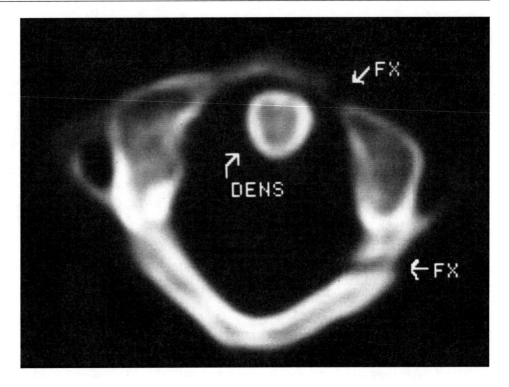

Occiput-C1 Injury

Atlanto-occipital injuries may occur during traumatic deliveries or major blunt trauma and imply an injury to the tectorial membrane and the alar ligaments (Fig. 5.8). Occiput-C1 injury or dislocation is rarely reported in surviving patients as it often results in lethal cervicomedullary cord damage [18]. Many occiput-C1 dislocations may spontaneously reduce and are initially unrecognized. These injuries are probably a result of sudden deceleration. The head is carried forward with a sudden craniovertebral dislocation and immediate spontaneous reduction and, hence, normal radiographic findings. Autopsy findings include disruption of the craniovertebral joints, spinal cord, and vertebral arteries.

For the rare individual who survives this injury, gentle reduction by positioning and minimal traction is recommended. Great care must be taken not to over-distract the injury site (Fig. 5.7). Halo fixation followed by posterior occipital cervical fusion is the definitive treatment. Chronic or late instability of occiput-C1 can be difficult to diagnose. Carefully controlled flexion-extension lateral views or reconstructed CT which allows calculation of the Powers ratio is helpful [39]. Fracture of an occipital condyle is infrequently reported and very difficult to diagnose [40].

Fractures of the Atlas

Fracture of the ring of C1, the so called Jefferson fracture, is not a common paediatric cervical fracture. The etiology is

an axial compression load applied to the head, transmitted through the lateral occipital condyles to the lateral masses of C1. The ring of C1 is usually broken at more than one site (Fig. 5.9). In children, isolated single fractures have been described, probably hinging on the synchondroses, which usually heal with immobilization [41]. Fractures have been reported through the synchondroses. As the lateral masses separate, the transverse atlantal ligament may rupture, or be avulsed (Fig. 5.10), and result in C1–C2 instability.

While plain radiography may show the fracture in certain cases, CT is far superior for visualizing the arch of C1 both acutely and in the follow-up period to assess healing (Fig. 5.9). Treatment should consist of a Minerva cast or halo immobilization. Surgery is rarely necessary to stabilize these fractures.

Odontoid Fractures

Odontoid fractures are among the most common cervical injuries in children, occurring at an average age of 4 years and are in reality growth plate injuries of the synchondroses (Fig. 5.11). The injury is frequently associated with head or facial trauma [42]. It may follow trivial head trauma. Children complaining of neck pain should always be radiographed. Clinically, they often resist attempts to extend the neck.

AP radiographs are often of little value since they may show only the normal synchondrotic line. The displacement or angulation may be seen only on the lateral view

Fig. 5.10 A 17-year-old who sustained a fracture of the ring of C1 from a direct blow to the skull. Note the avulsion of the lateral attachment of the transverse atlantal ligament (*arrow*)

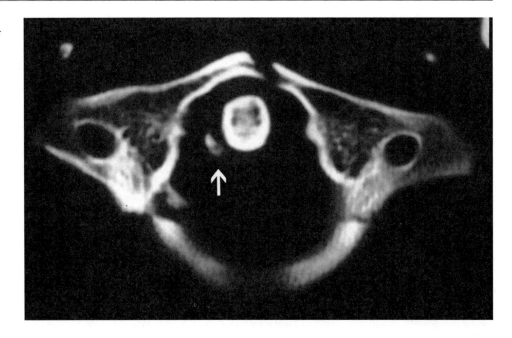

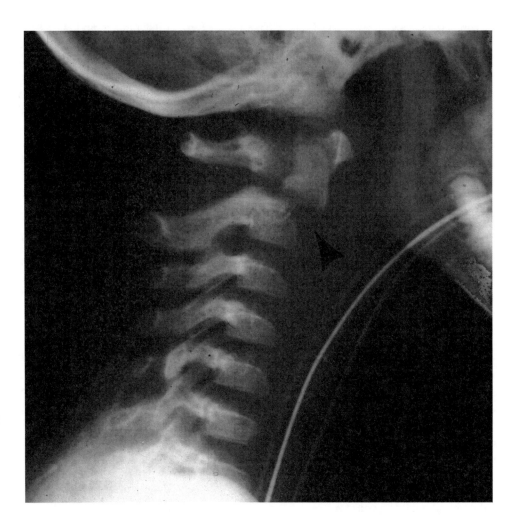

Fig. 5.11 Lateral radiograph of a young child with a fracture of the odontoid through the synchondrosis. This is a Salter–Harris type I injury and the periosteum is usually intact anteriorly

Fig. 5.12 Flexion and extension lateral radiographs of the cervical spine

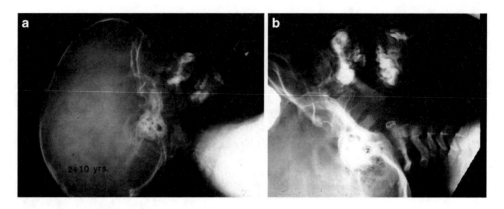

(Fig. 5.11). The displacement is usually anterior with the dens tilted posteriorly. However, posterior angulation of the odontoid process occurs in approximately 4% of normal children and should be interpreted with caution. Dynamic CT or MRI views in flexion and extension with lateral sagittal reconstruction are useful for evaluating instability [27, 35].

The diagnosis of odontoid injuries can be particularly difficult in children with underlying congenital and developmental cervical problems. In Morquio's syndrome, spondyloepiphyseal dysplasia, neurofibromatosis, osteogenesis imperfecta, and Down's syndrome dysplastic appearances of the odontoid make the diagnosis of fracture or instability problematic.

The rarity of complications and the generally good results in young children contrast sharply with complications such as non-union and the occasional late development of neurological sequelae in adults. Griffiths [43] suggested that an intact hinge of anterior periosteum might account for the apparent ease and stability of reduction in extension (Fig. 5.12) and by the early appearance of callus anteriorly.

We recommend reduction of acute odontoid fractures by recumbency in hyperextension as suggested by Sherk et al. [44], followed by a Minerva jacket or halo vest. These injuries should heal in 6 weeks. Following removal of the jacket or vest, healing should be confirmed by flexion-extension stress films. If there is no motion, then a soft collar should be worn for an additional 1–2 weeks. If reduction cannot be obtained by recumbency and hyperextension, then a head halter traction is suggested. Halo traction and, in rare cases, manipulation under general anesthesia should be reserved for those cases that are refractory to more conservative treatment [44]. Excellent long-term results can be expected without growth disturbance, indicating that the cartilage plate at the base of the odontoid contributes little to odontoid growth [5]. Connolly et al. [45] found that the odontoid fracture with anterior angulation does not need to be reduced and can be treated conservatively with excellent long-term follow-up. Many children with odontoid fractures were treated with halo vests for 3 months and did very well.

In the older child, odontoid fractures may cause instability and need stabilization with a screw [46]. Odent et al. [47] recently reported on fractures of the odontoid; 8 of 15 were secured in forward-facing car seats, yet sustained significant injuries in a motor vehicle accident.

Spondylolisthesis of C2 (Hangman's Fracture)

Bilateral spondylolisthesis of C2 has been occasionally reported in children from 6 to 18 months of age. The mechanism of injury is usually hyperextension and few are neurologically compromised [48]. Successful treatment can usually be accomplished through reduction by gentle positioning and immobilization in a halo or Minerva cast (Fig. 5.13). Surgery is only indicated for delayed or non-union union with instability. Traction is unnecessary and can produce a potentially dangerous neural distraction. (Hangman's fracture can occur with abused infants.)

Lower Cervical Injuries (C2–C7)

C2–C3 subluxation is one of the more difficult diagnostic problems in a child's injured neck. The radiographic findings may be similar to those of pseudosubluxation at C2–C3 (Fig. 5.5). The true nature of the lesion may only become apparent with time. It is important to correlate the radiographic picture with the clinical history and examination. A significant subluxation is more likely if the child sustained trauma followed by pain, spasm, limited motion, or tenderness. Persistence of symptoms after adequate conservative therapy is also suggestive of significant injury. Radiographically demonstrable abnormalities may be associated with the subluxation, such as ossification of the posterior longitudinal ligament, avulsion fractures of the tips of the spinous processes, compensatory lordosis, swan neck, or failure to correct the "subluxation" when the spine is placed in

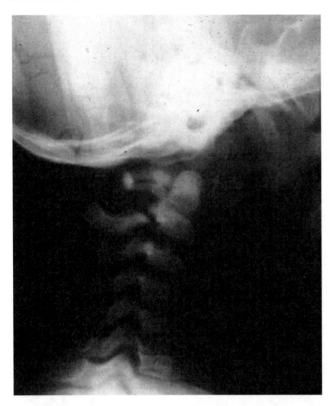

Fig. 5.13 Spondylolisthesis of C2 (hangman's fracture) in a 13-month-old boy. This can be treated with a Minerva cast in extension. From: Herzenberg JE, Hensinger RN. Pediatric cervical spine injuries. Trauma Quarterly 1989; 5:73–81. Used with permission

extension. Absent lordosis or reversal of lordosis may occur in normal subjects and is not always indicative of injury.

Injuries below C2 are less common in children than adults. Most reported injuries occur in teenagers in whom the cervical spine is near adult in configuration [17]. Many children with vertebral body flexion-compression fractures develop a persistent kyphotic deformity. Kyphosis cannot be prevented or cured by non-operative methods [49].

Hyperextension injuries to the lower cervical spine in children may result in physeal fracture, usually through the inferior vertebral endplate [7].

Many serious injuries below C3 are associated with ligamentous disruption and initially are unrecognized (Fig. 5.14). A ligamentous disruption causes gradual displacement of one segment on the other with secondary adaptive change making reduction difficult. If such lesions are suspected, regular follow-up is recommended with protection in an extension orthosis if necessary (Fig. 5.14). Posterior ligamentous disruption has limited potential for healing and if instability is documented the injury should be stabilized by posterior fusion (Fig. 5.15).

The management of teardrop fractures, facet dislocations, etc. in adolescents is similar to that in adults.

Immobilization

A variety of child-sized cervical stabilization devices are commercially available. They can be divided generally into rigid types made out of plastic and soft types made out of foam [50] (Fig. 5.16). While the rigid types perform better than soft foam in mechanical testing, even the best device allows 17° flexion, 19° extension, 4° rotation, and 6° lateral motion. To gain more control following an acute injury, Huerta et al. [51] recommend that these devices be supplemented with tape, bean bags, and other supports.

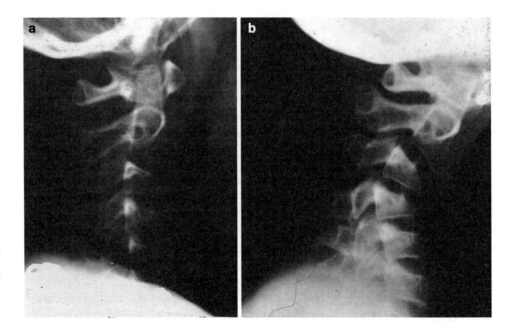

Fig. 5.14 (a) Lateral radiograph of a 14-year-old male who sustained a ligamentous injury of the cervical spine while playing football. (b) Four weeks later; note the marked cervical kyphosis at C3–C4

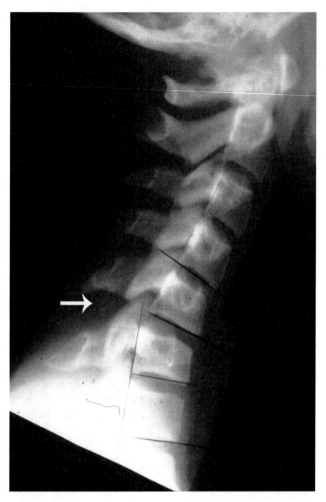

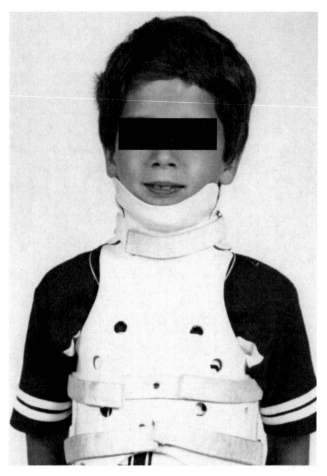

Fig. 5.16 A child immobilized in a SOMI brace

Fig. 5.15 Unstable ligamentous flexion injury in a teenage boy who fell backward while weight-lifting, striking the back of his head on a table. Note the kyphosis at C5–C6 and the small fleck of bone avulsed from the C5–C6 posterior facet joint (*arrow*).This injury would not heal adequately with immobilization alone. From: Herzenberg JE, Hensinger RN. Pediatric cervical spine injuries. Trauma Quarterly 1989; 5:73–81. Used with permission

The child with a cervical injury is at particular risk of further displacement during resuscitation. In a study of four patients with unstable cervical injuries who failed resuscitation in the emergency room, it was found that longitudinal axial traction during emergency intubation actually increased the deformity [52]. The authors recommended that intubation of trauma patients with suspected unstable cervical injuries prior to radiographic evaluation should be attempted first by the nasotracheal route rather than with axial traction and a standard laryngoscope. Cricothyroidotomy is another option.

While adults may be positioned safely supine on a flat backboard to immobilize the cervical spine, small children are different. Young children have disproportionately larger heads and are at risk of developing kyphosis and anterior translation of the upper cervical segment in an unstable fracture pattern (Fig. 5.17a and b). Curran et al. [53] showed

on lateral views of the cervical spine that 60% of the children were immobilized in over 5° of kyphosis and 37% had 10° or more. We must recognize the importance of transferring neck-injured patients safely in a neutral position: Children under 6 years should use a split mattress technique, elevating the thorax 2–4 cm and lowering the occiput (Fig. 5.17c and d). However, this immobilization protocol tends to reduce displaced fractures and makes their recognition more difficult [54]. Bosch et al. [20] do not recommend immobilization of patients with SCIWORA in order to reduce the risk of permanent neurological damage. However, the results of a meta-analysis indicate that external immobilization for 12 weeks seems slightly to reduce recurrence [55].

A plaster Minerva jacket is an excellent means of immobilizing the neck-injured child (Fig. 5.18). Thermoplastic bracing may be of value in the older child [50].

Skull tongs and halo devices can be used in the young child [56]. However, excessive pressure by halo pins or Crutchfield tongs can lead to skull perforation and brain abscess. Biomechanical and anatomical study of halo pin placement in children suggests the pins should be placed

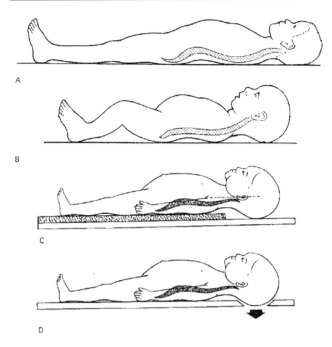

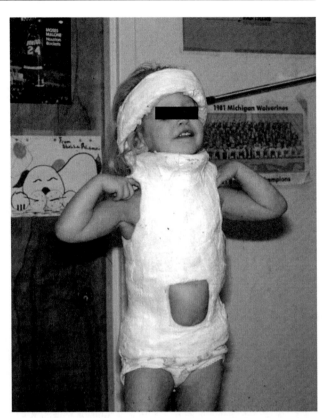

Fig. 5.17 (a) Adult immobilized on a standard backboard. (b) Young child on a standard backboard. The relatively large head forces the neck into a kyphotic position. (c) Young child on a modified backboard that has a double-mattress pad to raise the chest, obtaining safe supine cervical positioning. (d) Young child on a modified backboard that has a cut out to recess the occiput, obtaining safe supine cervical positioning. From: Herzenberg et al. [54]. Used with permission

Fig. 5.18 A 3-year-old with a fracture of the odontoid following 6 weeks immobilization in a Minerva cast

anterolaterally, posterolaterally, and perpendicular to the skull (Fig. 5.19). In the small child, a skull CT is needed to ensure there is sufficient bone for pin placement. A modified low-torque multiple pin technique allows the halo to be used in children as young as 7 months.

The halo body cast represents the most rigid form of external immobilization for cervical spine injuries in children. A halo vest does not limit motion sufficiently [56].

Surgical Stabilization

Fusion techniques in children differ little from those in the adult. Their spines fuse easily and it is prudent to expose only the relevant area [57]. Extending the dissection often leads to unwanted creeping fusion to the closely approximated adjacent laminae. Homologous bone grafting is not recommended. Stabler et al. [57] reported pseudarthrosis in six out of seven children aged 6–15 years following posterior wiring and fusion using cadaveric bone graft. Anterior cervical fusion in young children is not recommended for trauma.

Atlanto-axial arthrodesis in children is performed using techniques similar to the adult, but with smaller gauge

wire. In pre-operative planning, CT is essential to determine whether screw placement is feasible: Anderson et al. [58] recommend thin-cut (1 mm) CT scans with 2D sagittal and coronal reconstructions. Some type of stereotactic or other planning workstation helps to determine safe screw trajectories. C1–2 transarticular screws are the first choice whenever possible. They demonstrate resistance to all three planes of movement. This construct has provided excellent outcomes in adults and in a large number of children. The technique is not possible in 7–22% of patients because of variable location of the foramen transversarium and vulnerability of the vertebral artery [58–61]. Alternatives, which combine C1 lateral mass screws and C2 pars screws or C2 translaminar and subaxial lateral mass screws have been well less well studied (Anderson et al. [58]).

The vertebral arteries are locked in a groove on the upper surface of the posterior arch of C1 approximately 2 cm from the midline in the young child which leaves a narrow margin of safety. While halo immobilization may increase the rate of successful fusion, some use neither halo nor brace and report satisfactory results [58]. Many children who undergo posterior spine fusion for cervical fracture experience long-term mild chronic neck pain. McGrory and Klassen [62] reported 76% of children in a large series had excellent results after

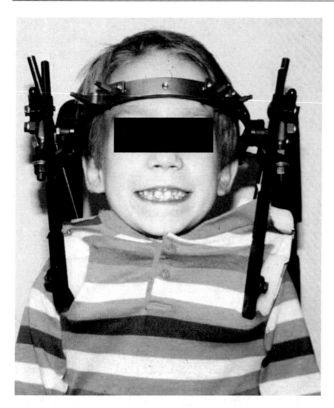

Fig. 5.19 Child immobilized in a halo cast following surgical stabilization of C1–C2 for instability secondary to Morquio's syndrome. Eight halo pins, four anteriorly and four posteriorly, help to distribute the forces on the skull over a larger area

neck fusion for fractures and dislocations. Complications included spontaneous extension of the fusion mass, continued pain at the iliac crest donor site, and superficial infection of the bone graft.

References

1. Cattell HS, Filtzer DL. Pseudosubluxation and other normal variations in the cervical spine in children. A study of one hundred and sixty children. J Bone Joint Surg Am 1965; 47: 1295–1309.
2. Avellino AM, Mann FA, Grady MS, et al. The misdiagnosis of acute cervical spine injuries and fractures in infants and children: the 12-year experience of a level I pediatric and adult trauma center. Childs Nerv Syst 2005; 21: 122–127.
3. Swischuk LE, Hayden CK Jr, Sarwar M. The dens-arch synchondrosis versus the hangman's fracture. Pediatr Radiol 1979; 8: 100–102.
4. Fielding JW, Hensinger RN, Hawkins RJ. Os odontoideum. J Bone Joint Surg Am 1980; 62: 376–383.
5. Sherk HH, Schut L, Lane JM. Fractures and dislocations of the cervical spine in children. Orthop Clin North Am 1976; 7: 593–604.
6. Caffey J. The whiplash shaken infant syndrome: manual shaking by the extremities with whiplash-induced intracranial and intraocular bleedings, linked with residual permanent brain damage and mental retardation. Pediatrics 1974; 54: 396–403.
7. Lawson JP, Ogden JA, Bucholz RW, et al. Physeal injuries of the cervical spine. J Pediatr Orthop 1987; 7: 428–435.
8. Fielding JW, Cochran GB, Lawsing JF 3rd, et al. Tears of the transverse ligament of the atlas. A clinical and biomechanical study. J Bone Joint Surg Am 1974; 56: 1683–1691.
9. Pennecot GF, Gouraud D, Hardy JR, et al. Roentgenographical study of the stability of the cervical spine in children. J Pediatr Orthop 1984; 4: 346–352.
10. Burke SW, French HG, Roberts JM, et al. Chronic atlanto-axial instability in Down syndrome. J Bone Joint Surg Am 1985; 67: 1356–1360.
11. McRae DL. The significance of abnormalities of the cervical spine. Am J Roentgenol 1960; 84: 3–25.
12. Steel HH. Anatomical and mechanical consideration of the atlanto-axial articulation. Proceedings of the American Orthopaedic Association. J Bone Joint Surg 1968; 50A: 1481–1482.
13. Swischuk LE. Anterior displacement of C2 in children: physiologic or pathologic. Radiology 1977; 122: 759–763.
14. White AA 3rd, Johnson RM, Panjabi MM, et al. Biomechanical analysis of clinical stability in the cervical spine. Clin Orthop 1975; 85–96.
15. Wholey MH, Bruwer AJ, Baker HL Jr. The lateral roentgenogram of the neck; with comments on the atlanto-odontoid-basion relationship. Radiology 1958; 71: 350–356.
16. Pang D. Spinal cord injury without radiographic abnormality in children, 2 decades later. Neurosurg 2004; 55: 1325–1342; discussion 1342–1323.
17. Hause M, Hoshino R, Omata S, et al. Cervical spine injuries in children Clin Orthop 1977; 129: 172–176.
18. Brown RL, Brunn MA, Garcia VF. Cervical spine injuries in children: a review of 103 patients treated consecutively at a level 1 pediatric trauma center. J Pediatr Surg 2001; 36: 1107–1114.
19. Eleraky MA, Theodore N, Adams M, et al. Pediatric cervical spine injuries: report of 102 cases and review of the literature. J Neurosurg 2000; 92: 12–17.
20. Bosch PP, Vogt MT, Ward WT. Pediatric spinal cord injury without radiographic abnormality (SCIWORA): the absence of occult instability and lack of indication for bracing. Spine 2002; 27: 2788–2800.
21. Kokoska ER, Keller MS, Rallo MC, et al. Characteristics of pediatric cervical spine injuries. J Pediatr Surg 2001; 36: 100–105.
22. Carreon LY, Glassman SD, Campbell MJ. Pediatric spine fractures: a review of 137 hospital admissions. J Spinal Disord Tech 2004; 17:477–482.
23. Furnival RA, Street KA, Schunk JE. Too many pediatric trampoline injuries. Pediatrics 1999; 103: e57.
24. Gonzalez RP, Fried PO, Bukhalo M, et al. Role of clinical examination in screening for blunt cervical spine injury. J Am Coll Surg 1999; 189: 152–157.
25. Rachesky I, Boyce WT, Duncan B, et al. Clinical prediction of cervical spine injuries in children. Radiographic abnormalities. Am J Dis Child 1987; 141: 199–201.
26. Berne JD, Velmahos GC, El-Tawil Q, et al. Value of complete cervical helical computed tomographic scanning in identifying cervical spine injury in the unevaluable blunt trauma patient with multiple injuries: a prospective study. J Trauma 1999; 47: 896–902; discussion 902–893.
27. Sanchez B, Waxman K, Jones T, et al. Cervical spine clearance in blunt trauma: evaluation of a computed tomography-based protocol. J Trauma 2005; 59: 179–183.
28. Woodring JH, Lee C. The role and limitations of computed tomographic scanning in the evaluation of cervical trauma. J Trauma 1992; 33: 698–708.
29. Tan E, Schweitzer ME, Vaccaro L, et al. Is computed tomography of nonvisualized C7-T1 cost-effective? J Spinal Disord 1999; 12: 472–476.

30. Pang D, Wilberger JE Jr. Spinal cord injury without radiographic abnormalities in children. J Neurosurg 1982; 57: 114–129.

31. Yngve DA, Harris WP, Herndon WA, et al. Spinal cord injury without osseous spine fracture. J Pediatr Orthop 1988; 8: 153–159.

32. Osenbach RK, Menezes AH. Spinal cord injury without radiographic abnormality in children. Pediatr Neurosci 1989; 15: 168–174; discussion 175.

33. Katzberg RW, Benedetti PF, Drake CM, et al. Acute cervical spine injuries: prospective MR imaging assessment at a level 1 trauma center. Radiology 1999; 213: 203–212.

34. Buldini B, Amigoni A, Faggin R, et al. Spinal cord injury without radiographic abnormalities. Eur J Pediatr 2006; 165: 108–111.

35. Dare AO, Dias MS, Li V. Magnetic resonance imaging correlation in pediatric spinal cord injury without radiographic abnormality. J Neurosurg 2002; 97: 3 3–39.

36. Stern WE, Rand RW. Birth injuries to the spinal cord: a report of 2 cases and review of the literature. Am J Obstet Gynecol 1959; 78: 498–512.

37. Caird MS, Reddy S, Ganley TJ, et al. Cervical spine fracture-dislocation birth injury: prevention, recognition, and implications for the orthopaedic surgeon. J Pediatr Orthop 2005; 25: 484–486.

38. Swischuk LE. Spine and spinal cord trauma in the battered child syndrome. Radiology 1969; 92: 733–738.

39. Powers B, Miller MD, Kramer RS, et al. Traumatic anterior atlanto-occipital dislocation. Neurosurg 1979; 4: 12–17.

40. Cottalorda J, Allard D, Dutour N. Fracture of the occipital condyle. J Pediatr Orthop B 1996; 5: 61–63.

41. Reilly CW, Leung F. Synchondrosis fracture in a pediatric patient. Can J Surg 2005; 48: 158–159.

42. Nachemson A. Fracture of the odontoid process of the axis. A clinical study based on 26 cases. Acta Orthop Scan 1960; 20: 185–217.

43. Griffiths SC. Fracture of odontoid process in children. J Pediatr Surg 1972; 7: 680–683.

44. Sherk HH, Nicholson JT, Chung SM. Fractures of the odontoid process in young children. J Bone Joint Surg Am 1978; 60: 921–924.

45. Connolly B, Emery D, Armstrong D. The odontoid synchondrotic slip: an injury unique to young children. Pediatr Radiol 1995; 25 Suppl 1:S129–133.

46. Morandi X, Hanna A, Hamlat A, et al. Anterior screw fixation of odontoid fractures. Surg Neurol 1999; 51: 236–240.

47. Odent T, Langlais J, Glorion C, et al. Fractures of the odontoid process: a report of 15 cases in children younger than 6 years. J Pediatr Orthop 1999; 19: 51–54.

48. Kleinman PK, Shelton YA. Hangman's fracture in an abused infant: imaging features. Pediatr Radiol 1997; 27: 776–777.

49. Schwarz N, Genelin F, Schwarz AF. Post-traumatic cervical kyphosis in children cannot be prevented by non-operative methods. Injury 1994; 25: 173–175.

50. Millington PJ, Ellingsen JM, Hauswirth BE, et al. Thermoplastic Minerva body jacket—a practical alternative to current methods of cervical spine stabilization. A clinical report. Phys Ther 1987; 67: 223–225.

51. Huerta C, Griffith R, Joyce SM. Cervical spine stabilization in pediatric patients: evaluation of current techniques. Ann Emerg Med 1987; 16: 1121–1126.

52. Bivins HG, Ford S, Bezmalinovic Z, et al. The effect of axial traction during orotracheal intubation of the trauma victim with an unstable cervical spine. Ann Emerg Med 1988; 17: 25–29.

53. Curran C, Dietrich AM, Bowman MJ, et al. Pediatric cervical-spine immobilization: achieving neutral position? J Trauma. 1995; 39: 729–732.

54. Herzenberg JE, Hensinger RN, Dedrick DK, et al. Emergency transport and positioning of young children who have an injury of the cervical spine. The standard backboard may be hazardous. J Bone Joint Surg Am 1989; 71: 15–22.

55. Launay F, Leet AI, Sponseller PD. Pediatric spinal cord injury without radiographic abnormality: a meta-analysis. Clin Orthop 2005: 166–170.

56. Letts M, Kaylor D, Gouw G. A biomechanical analysis of halo fixation in children. J Bone Joint Surg Br 1988; 70: 277–279.

57. Stabler CL, Eismont FJ, Brown MD, et al. Failure of posterior cervical fusions using cadaveric bone graft in children. J Bone Joint Surg Am 1985; 67: 371–375.

58. Anderson RC, Ragel BT, Mocco J, et al. Selection of a rigid internal fixation construct for stabilization at the craniovertebral junction in pediatric patients. J Neurosurg 2007; 107: 36–42.

59. Brockmeyer DL, York JE, Apfelbaum RI. Anatomical suitability of C1–2 transarticular screw placement in pediatric patients. J Neurosurg 2000; 92: 7–11.

60. Igarashi T, Kikuchi S, Sato K, et al. Anatomic study of the axis for surgical planning of transarticular screw fixation. Clin Orthop 2003:162–166.

61. Madawi AA, Casey AT, Solanki GA, et al. Radiological and anatomical evaluation of the atlantoaxial transarticular screw fixation technique. J Neurosurg 1997; 86: 961–968.

62. McGrory BJ, Klassen RA. Arthrodesis of the cervical spine for fractures and dislocations in children and adolescents. A long-term follow-up study. J Bone Joint Surg Am 1994; 76: 1606–1616.

Chapter 6

Fractures of the Thoracic and Lumbar Spine

Robert N. Hensinger and Clifford L. Craig

General and Basic Principles

Injuries of the thoracic and lumbar spine in children are rare. The potential for continued growth, the presence of healthy disc tissue, the elasticity of the soft tissues, and well-mineralized bone distinguish these injuries from those in the adult. The immature spine has the capacity to remodel the vertebral body, but not the posterior elements. Restoration of height of a compressed vertebra is partly due to the hypervascularity of the reparative response and partly due to apophyseal stimulation. This probably accounts for the infrequent occurrence of kyphosis in children with multiple compression fractures.

The development of the thoracolumbar spine in children is more straightforward than that of the cervical spine. One should be aware of the following: (i) an increased cartilage to bone ratio; (ii) the presence of the ring apophysis; and (iii) hyperelasticity. In the newborn and in early childhood, the vertebrae are largely cartilaginous, and radiographically the intervertebral spaces appear widened in relation to the vertebral bodies (Fig. 6.1). With aging, the ossification centers enlarge and the cartilage to bone ratio gradually reverses. The vertebral apophyses are secondary centers of ossification that develop in the cartilaginous endplates located at the superior and inferior surfaces of the vertebral bodies. They are thicker at their periphery than at the center, and thus appear as a ring with early ossification. They are first seen radiologically between the eighth and the twelfth years and normally fuse with the vertebral bodies by the twenty-first year. They may be confused with avulsion fractures. The vertebral apophysis is equivalent to the epiphysis of a long bone and is separated from the vertebral body (the metaphysis) by a narrow cartilaginous physis. Vertical growth of the vertebrae occurs equally at the top and the bottom.

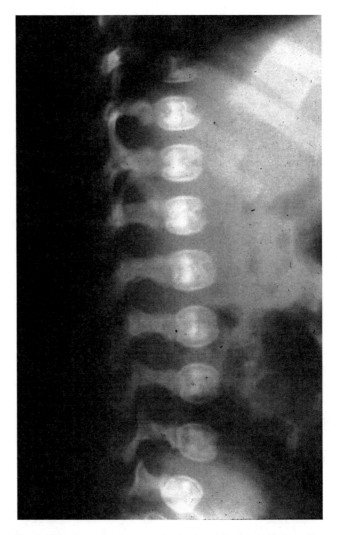

Fig. 6.1 Radiograph of a normal spine in a 10-week-old infant. The superior and inferior vertebral endplates, the vertebral apophyses, are cartilaginous. Thus, the apparent widening of the intervertebral spaces is relative to the ossific portion of the vertebrae. The anterior and posterior notching of the walls of the vertebral body is due to the normal vascular channels and may be confused with fracture

In the infant, on the lateral radiograph, horizontal conical or "notch" shadows of decreased density are seen extending

R.N. Hensinger (✉)
Department of Orthopaedic Surgery, University of Michigan, Ann Arbor, MI, USA

inward from the anterior and posterior walls of the vertebral bodies, which may be confused with fracture [1] (Fig. 6.1). The posterior notch results from an actual indentation in the posterior vertebra wall at the point of entrance and emergence of the posterior arteries and veins. This indentation is present in all vertebrae and at all ages [1]. In the infant, the anterior conical shadow is usually more obvious than the posterior and represents a large sinusoidal space within the vertebra [1]. It disappears, usually in the first year of life, as the anterior and lateral walls of the vertebral body ossify.

Leventhal [2] demonstrated that in the infant and young child the cervical vertebral bodies function as a series of elastic cartilages which can be stretched up to 5 cm without disruption, while the less elastic cervical spinal cord tolerates only 6 mm. This differential elasticity probably accounts for the frequent occurrence in the young child of spinal cord damage without radiological evidence of bony injury, both in the cervical and in the thoracolumbar spine [3–9]. Magnetic resonance imaging (MRI) has helped to confirm spinal cord lesions in children with traumatic paraplegia from stretching or blunt injury following dislocation and spontaneous reduction or vascular compromise [9, 10].

By 8–10 years, the bony thoracolumbar spine has approached the biomechanical properties of the adult and fracture patterns are very similar, with the exception of late-developing progressive spinal deformity. Paralytic scoliosis occurs in virtually all children who sustain a complete spinal cord injury prior to the adolescent growth spurt age [11]. Possible causes include injury to the vertebral body growth plate as well as muscle imbalance, spasticity, and the influence of gravity [11–13]. As in the neck, thoracic laminectomy increases the likelihood of a progressive kyphosis by 36% [14]. Disc space narrowing and spontaneous interbody fusion after injury are uncommon in children, as the healthy intervertebral discs typically transmit the force to the vertebral bodies [13]. Thus, there is a stronger case for initial conservative management of the spine in children than in adults since up to two-thirds have a stable spine.

Incidence

Childhood spinal fractures are uncommon (2–5% of all spinal injuries [3, 6, 15–17]). While most occur in the cervical spine, significant and disabling injuries take place in the thoracic and lumbar regions. In the series reported by Reddy et al. [18], the thoracic spine was more commonly injured than the lumbar region. The thoracolumbar and cervicothoracic junctions were at risk. There was no relationship to gender or mechanism of injury. The mechanism of injury varies with the age of the patient. Neonates are more prone to cervical than to dorsal or lumbar spine injury [2, 19]. Occasionally, infant spinal injuries are due to

child abuse [20, 21]. The young child in the first decade is more often involved in pedestrian/motor vehicle injuries, as a passenger in a car, or in falls from heights [5, 8, 22–26]. In the second decade, spinal injuries are often (44%) the result of sports and recreational activities, such as tobogganing, cycling, and motorcycling [4, 27–29]. In the United States, American football injuries are the leading cause of sports-related injuries (38%) [24]. Motor vehicle accidents account for 37% of injuries [6]. It is believed that as many as 50% of children who have mild vertebral injuries are never admitted to the hospital and the reported statistics are therefore skewed toward the more severely injured [6, 30]. One should be particularly suspicious of the multiply injured child, as it is easy to overlook significant vertebral fractures. The increased elasticity of children means that the injuring force is transmitted over many segments, with multiple vertebral fractures the rule [13, 17, 25, 31] (Fig. 6.2).

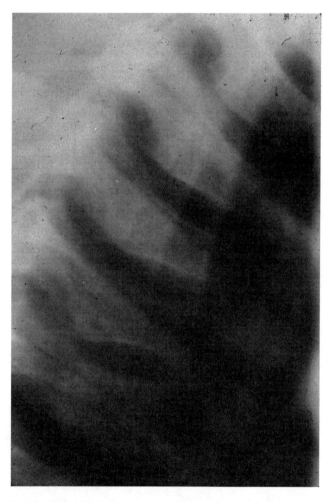

Fig. 6.2 Radiograph of a 5-year-old girl who sustained compression fractures of three vertebrae from a sledging accident. Note reversal of the normally convex endplate, beaking, and wedging of the vertebral bodies. Overlapping of the spongiosum may appear as increased density. The child was asymptomatic within 6 weeks, and complete restitution of the vertebral height can be expected

Similarly, innocuous-appearing fractures of the lumbar or thoracic transverse processes are often associated with serious injury to the abdomen (20%), particularly the spleen and the liver, to the pelvis and urinary tract, or to the chest [24, 32–34].

Mechanisms of Injury

The three-column system described by Denis [35, 36] permits vertebral injuries to be divided into four major types (Fig. 6.3):

1. *Compression fracture*: failure of the anterior column with an intact middle column.
2. *Burst fracture*: failure under compression (usually axial) of both the anterior and the middle columns.

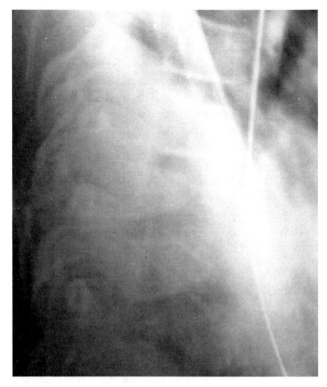

Fig. 6.4 Severe fracture dislocation of the thoracic spine in a 13-year-old male. The patient crashed in a motocross accident at a high rate of speed and was thrown 6 m. Complete paraplegia at the scene. MRI showed complete transection of the spinal cord. The thoracic fracture was reduced and stabilized with internal fixation

3. *Seat-belt fracture*: compression injury of the anterior column with distraction of the middle and posterior columns through either bony or ligamentous elements.
4. *Fracture dislocation*: all three columns fail in compression with rotation and shear of the anterior column, distraction and shear of the middle column, and distraction with rotation and shear of the posterior column (Fig. 6.4).

Compression

Compression injuries due to hyperflexion are more common than distraction, shear, or subluxation/dislocation injuries [26, 37]. In the immature spine, the intact disc is more resistant to vertical compression than is the vertebral body. Roaf [38] experimentally loaded the vertebrae vertically with a slow increase in pressure and demonstrated that the major distortion was a bulge in the vertebral endplate, with only a slight change in the annulus and no alteration in the shape of the nucleus pulposus. He observed that the bulging of the endplate caused the blood to be squeezed out of the cancellous bone. This led him to suggest that the blood in the spongiosa was a major shock-absorbing mechanism.

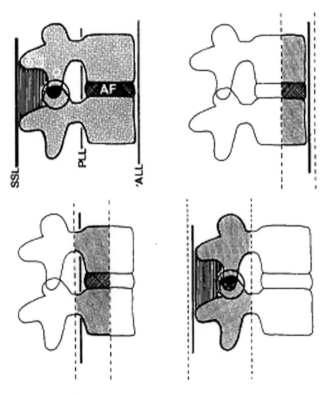

Fig. 6.3 Illustration of the anterior middle and posterior columns after Denis. Supraspinous ligament (SSL), posterior longitudinal ligament (PLL), anterior longitudinal ligament (ALL), and annulus fibrosus (AF). (1) The anterior column includes the anterior longitudinal ligament, the anterior portion of the annulus fibrosis, and the anterior portion of the vertebral body. (2) The middle column is formed by the posterior longitudinal ligament, the posterior annulus fibrosis, and the posterior wall of the vertebral body. (3) The posterior column includes the posterior bony complex, the posterior arch, the posterior ligamentous complex [supraspinous ligament, infraspinous ligament (ISL), capsule (Cl)], and the ligamentum flavum (LF). From: Denis [35]. Used with permission

With greater force, the endplate broke and the nuclear material ruptured into the vertebral body. The two vertebrae moved closer together with a diminution of the disc space (Fig. 6.5). Thus, when a child's spine is hyperflexed, such as during tobogganing or tubing, the blood is squeezed from the vertebra, the shock-absorbing properties are decreased, and less force is required to cause a vertebral injury [27, 28] (Fig. 6.6).

In older patients, Roaf [38] found that the nucleus is no longer fluid, and compression forces are transmitted through the annulus. Applied pressure then led to either tearing of the annulus with general collapse of the vertebrae due to buckling of the sides or a marginal plateau fracture [38]. An even greater or more rapidly applied force caused a bursting injury, similar to that seen in adults [39]. Unstable burst fractures are accompanied by posterior column injuries, such as the seat-belt injuries, resulting from flexion and distraction [40]. Roaf also found that the child's disc has more turgor and is capable of transmitting force through several levels [6, 29, 31, 38, 41]. Clinically, the multiple compression fractures (50–75%) typical of childhood usually occur from the mid-thoracic to the mid-lumbar areas [17, 26, 37, 41]. Roaf [38] noted that, when the immature spine is compressed, the vertebral body always breaks before the normal disc gives way, unless there was pre-injury to the annulus: then it balloons like a tire. This is supported clinically as there are few children reported with posterior herniated discs and these follow significant loading injuries, such as weight lifting and gymnastics [42]. Occasionally, a calcified disc may herniate [43, 44].

Distraction and Shear

Aufdemaur studied children killed by violent injuries (e.g., being hit by a car) and found that their fractures were primarily of the shear type [15]. Typically, the injury did not cause rupture of the intervertebral disc, but rather the vertebrae fractured through the cartilaginous endplate apophysis (Fig. 6.7). Infrequently, children may have a flexion–rotation injury combined with compression, which leads to a shearing injury and spondylolisthesis (Fig. 6.8).

Slipped Vertebral Apophysis

Several authors have described patients, usually adolescent boys, with traumatic displacement of a lumbar vertebral ring apophysis into the spinal canal with associated disc protrusion [45–49] (Fig. 6.9). Most were from the postero-inferior rim of L4 and less commonly from the inferior rim of L3 or L5. The age group and circumstances suggest that the vertebral endplate may be more susceptible during the phase of rapid growth, analogous to the slipped capital femoral epiphysis [50]. Indeed, acute and chronic forms have been described and the problem is often erroneously diagnosed as a herniated disc [51, 52]. Dietemann et al. [51] in their series noted a high association (38%) with lumbar Scheuermann's disease, and a pre-existing marginal Schmorl's node may weaken the edge and lead to the slip [52] (Fig. 6.9a).

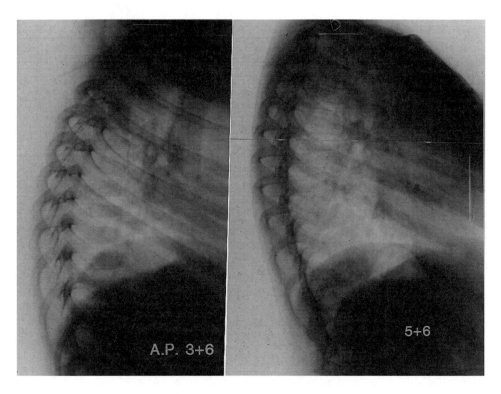

Fig. 6.5 Left: Radiograph of a 3½-year-old girl who was involved in a fall, sustaining multiple compression fractures. Right: The same patient at age 5½. Radiograph demonstrates remodeling of this injury. She was treated conservatively, is asymptomatic, and returned to near-normal vertebral height

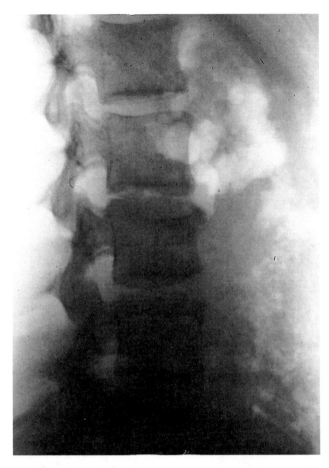

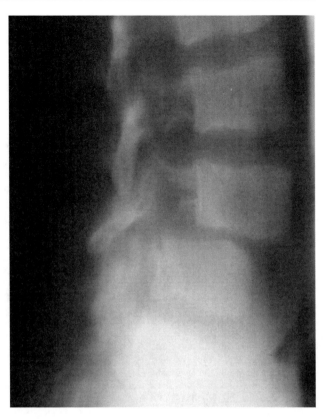

Fig. 6.6 Radiograph of a 15-year-old girl who sustained an injury to the vertebral body from tobogganing, demonstrating a fracture of the apophyseal ring and displacement anteriorly. From: Rockwood CA, Wilkin KE, Beaty JH, eds. Fractures in Children, Volume 3, 4th Edition, Philadelphia: Lippincott-Raven, 1996. Used with permission

Fig. 6.8 Traumatic spondylolysis with severe disruption of the pedicle and the facet. Lateral laminagraphic radiograph of a 13-year-old boy scout who sustained this lumbar fracture when a tree fell directly across his back during a storm. Lateral view demonstrates a shear-type injury with a fracture dislocation of L4–L5. From: Rockwood CA, Wilkin KE, Beaty JH, eds. Fractures in Children, Volume 3, 4th Edition, Philadelphia: Lippincott-Raven, 1996. Used with permission

Fig. 6.7 Distraction injury: Radiograph of the newborn with complete disruption at T3–T4. The patient was a breech delivery with cephalopelvic disproportion, leading to a difficult extraction. (**a**) Anteroposterior view. (**b**) Lateral view, demonstrating that the fracture is through the cartilage endplate. The child is totally paraplegic at that level and also has paralysis of the right hemidiaphragm. From: Rockwood CA, Wilkin KE, Beaty JH, eds. Fractures in Children, Volume 3, 4th Edition, Philadelphia: Lippincott-Raven, 1996. Used with permission

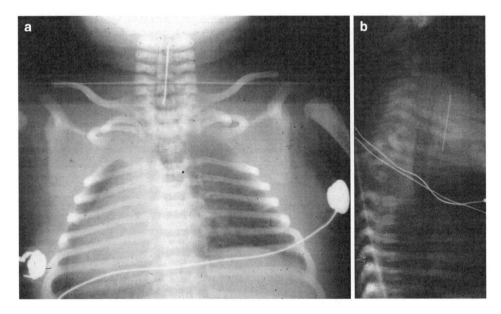

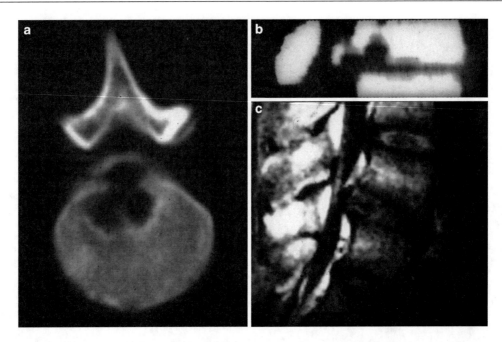

Fig. 6.9 Slipped vertebral apophysis. A 13-year-old with back pain, tight hamstrings, and symptoms suggestive of spinal stenosis. (**a**) CT scan demonstrating a Schmorl's node formation and a fracture of the apophysis with subluxation into the spinal canal. (**b**) CT reconstruction of the same lesion. (**c**) MRI demonstrating slipping of the vertebral apophysis as well as the intervertebral disc with encroachment of the spinal canal. Lateral radiograph of the lumbosacral junction demonstrates Schmorl's node formation and bony changes in the posterior portion of the apophysis of L4. From: Rockwood CA, Wilkin KE, Beaty JH, eds. Fractures in Children, Volume 3, 4th Edition, Philadelphia: Lippincott-Raven, 1996. Used with permission

Radiographically, all cases demonstrate a small bony fragment (edge of the vertebral endplate) within the spinal canal and a large anterior extradural impression or complete block on MRI from the radiolucent protruded disc [50] (Fig. 6.9c). Computed tomography (CT) has proven excellent in confirming the diagnosis [51, 52]. The onset is usually acute after an injury such as during weight lifting or shoveling [50]. The children have the signs and symptoms of a central herniated disc, with muscle weakness, absent reflexes, and limited straight-leg raising [37]. Later findings are similar to spinal stenosis. Laminectomy and decompression by surgical removal of the disc and bony ridge give excellent relief of symptoms [50, 52]. Surgical removal of the disc alone is not sufficient to relieve nerve root impingement [50].

Chance Fractures in Children

The pathomechanics of this injury was first described by Smith and Kaufer [53]. They reviewed lumbar spine injuries associated with seat belts and described the mechanism as forward flexion over a lap belt, producing distraction of the posterior vertebral elements and anterior compression. This injury was previously uncommon in children [54]. As rear seats continue often to have lap belts only, the injury appears to be increasing in children [55]. The fracture levels are primarily the lumbar spine, usually between L1 and L3, but can occur at L4 (Fig. 6.10). In children, the injury is more likely in the mid-lumbar spine, whereas in adults, the injury is at the thoracolumbar junction, which may be due to their having a higher center of gravity [56]. In the rear seats, adult lap belts do not provide protection equivalent to child safety or booster seats. In the absence of this child safety equipment, a shoulder harness should be considered [32]. In adults with this injury, there has been a high association with intra-abdominal pathology (50%), and in children, it would appear even higher [32, 55] (Fig. 6.11). Ecchymosis in a lap-belt distribution should always alert the examiner to look for a chance fracture [32]. In the series by Gumley et al. [57], the abdominal injuries were so severe that they dominated the early clinical picture and the spinal fracture was detected late. The reverse has also been reported. Bilateral facet dislocations are slightly more common than fractures through the lamina. In Betz et al. reported 30–50% of children with lap-belt injuries had associated retroperitoneal injuries [58].

Agran et al. [59] divided the 191 children who were wearing seat belts when they were involved in motor vehicle accidents into the following three groups:

1. Infants and toddlers (0–3 years): these children had proportionally larger heads and higher centers of gravity

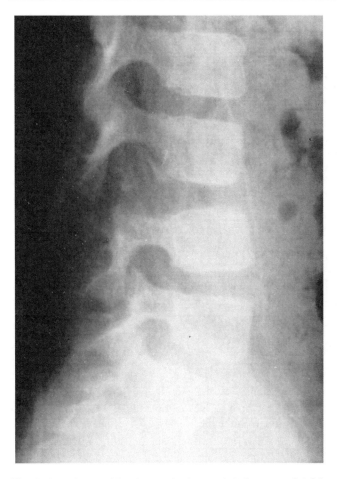

Fig. 6.10 A 3-year-old male sustained a seat-belt fracture at L1–L2 as a restrained backseat passenger. The lateral view demonstrates spreading and angulation of the spinous process and vertebral bodies, suggesting posterior ligamentous disruption similar to the chance fracture in the adult

and sustained injuries to chest and abdominal organs. He noted that children tend to undergo a rotational movement and easily become airborne and move headfirst to the side of the impact.

2. Middle-aged children (4–9 years): the center of gravity is closer to the umbilicus. The iliac crests are not adequately developed and the seat belt tends to slide up and lie over the abdomen.

3. Adolescents (10–14 years): the physique is similar to the adult.

Routine lateral views of the spine are best for making this diagnosis. The CT scan may not reveal the presence of this injury due to limitations in detecting horizontal fractures and dislocations in the axial plane [56]. Distraction and apophyseal injuries are notoriously difficult to exclude with CT scans [60]. Reverse hyperextension injuries of the lumbar spine have been described in children [61]. Similarly, a

fracture through the posterior elements alone without lumbar fracture has been reported in children and adults [22].

Neurological Injury

Between 13 and 20% of all spinal cord injuries occur in children, with higher frequencies in the young child and males predominating (2:1) [6, 26, 62]. In the cervical spine the vertebral column in the young child is more elastic than the spinal cord itself [2]. An infantile spinal canal can be stretched 5 cm, and the cervical cord only 6 mm. Similarly, many children have been reported, particularly those under 10 who have a significant spinal cord injury without observable radiographic injury (SCIWORA) [3–6, 8, 9, 12, 16, 17, 63–65]. MRI has been very helpful to identify the site and extent of the lesion and may show acute hemorrhage or edema of the spinal cord [9, 10, 66, 67].

There are two incidence peaks: (i) those younger than 10 years and (ii) teenagers. In the young child, the lesion is more often at the cervicothoracic junction [9] and the paraplegia is more likely to be permanent. The teenager is more likely to have an incomplete neurological deficit that resolves or improves [17, 62]. Choi et al. [10] reviewed patients with delayed onset of paraplegia (2 h to 4 days) and suggested that this group represents a vascular insult to the spinal cord. The location was typically at the midportion of the thoracic spine (watershed area) and usually associated with a blow to the chest or the abdomen, resulting in shock or profound hypotension from a ruptured spleen or retroperitoneal hematoma. This generally results in complete and permanent paraplegia. The MRI is helpful in delineating the lesion and laminectomy was of no benefit [10, 66].

In the older child, vertebral fracture is the most common cause of neurological injury, and in the majority (83%) a bony injury can be identified radiologically [6]. Fracture dislocations are more commonly the cause of spinal cord injury, usually at the thoracolumbar junction (36%) and the remainder between T4 and L2 [6, 17, 25, 26, 31, 64].

Symptoms and Signs

Several problems peculiar to children may result in diagnostic errors unless a careful clinical and radiographic examination is performed. Failure to recognize paralysis represents the most serious error. An unresponsive or comatose child should be considered to have a spinal injury until proven otherwise. In one study, the most common extraspinal injury was a head injury [62]. Determining paralysis or the extent of paralysis may prove difficult in an uncooperative child.

Fig. 6.11 Seat-belt injury at L1–L2. (**a**) Lateral and (**b**) AP view in a 7-year-old male. Severe disruption of the soft tissue posteriorly with forward translation of L1 on L2. This injury was associated with traumatic paraplegia (complete) and severe abdominal injuries (bowel, pancreas). Many children with seat-belt fractures have serious abdominal injuries, which can be life threatening. From: Rockwood CA, Wilkin KE, Beaty JH, eds. Fractures in Children, Volume 3, 4th Edition, Philadelphia: Lippincott-Raven, 1996. Used with permission

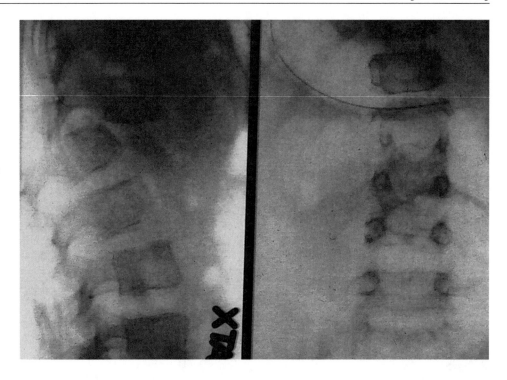

Gross flexion or reflex withdrawal of the limbs may mislead one into thinking that voluntary movement is present.

Stimulation and handling may produce crying and can lead the physician to erroneously assume that sensation is intact. Serial observation over a period of time may be necessary to determine the true neurological status of the patient. The diagnosis of birth injuries of the spinal cord should be suspected in a floppy infant or a child with a nonprogressive neurological lesion following a difficult delivery. The single most important finding is the demonstration of a sensory level. In the older child, pain and tenderness over the spine are usually present, similar to the adult. Inability to walk and muscle spasm are often present with unstable injuries of the spine.

Imaging Features

The radiological appearance depends on the force and mechanism of injury. Compression due to hyperflexion is the most common injury and can range from slight flattening of the normally convex endplates to frank wedging of the vertebrae [16] (Fig. 6.2). Hegenbarth and Ebel [25] suggested a classification of compression fractures in children based on the appearance: (i) wedge shaped or (ii) beak shaped with upper or lower prominent anterior contours. Both types may be asymmetrical on the sagittal view as well as the frontal view. There may be a zone of increased density in the vertebral body due to compression and overlapping of the spongiosa

[25, 26]. In the infant, anterior and posterior notching of the vertebral bodies due to the normal vascular channels may be confused with fracture [1] (Fig. 6.1). Multiply damaged vertebrae are the rule, but clinically observable kyphosis is uncommon unless there is a fracture dislocation [25] (Fig. 6.10). The thoracic spine is often difficult to evaluate with conventional radiographs and careful attention should be paid to this area. CT may be helpful [18]. True fracture lines are seldom seen in the young child prior to puberty (Fig. 6.6). Damage to a vertebral endplate is not likely to be severe enough to cause cessation of growth [40]. Rarely is there an avulsed vertebral corner as might be seen in the adult [26] (Fig. 6.6). With greater force, the endplate ruptures and the disc is extruded into the vertebral body, forming a Schmorl's node, commonly in the lower thoracic and upper lumbar vertebrae [23]. Typical adult fracture patterns are less commonly seen, such as complete fracture of the vertebral body and fracture dislocation and subluxation of the facets. As with the adult, CT and sagittal reconstruction are more accurate in detecting posterior arch fractures and assessing bony fragments and narrowing of the spinal canal [18, 60, 68–70]. Positioning is important, particularly in the injured child. The tomographic cuts must be at right angles to the vertebrae or the lesion will be confused with a pseudo-fracture [68]. MRI is better at detecting injuries to the soft tissue, such as ligaments, intervertebral disc, or spinal cord, and impingement of the spinal cord by the intervertebral disc or epidural hematoma [60, 66, 70, 71]. Sledge et al. [60] conclude that MRI is the imaging modality of choice in patients with thoracolumbar injuries because it can

accurately classify injury to bones and ligaments and because the spinal cord patterns as determined by MRI have predictive value. The younger the patient and the more the vertebral column is composed of cartilage, the harder it is to characterize fully a spinal injury by radiographs and CT scan. Sledge et al. [60] found that posterior fractures were more difficult to rule out by MRI. They missed two that were found on CT. MRI is helpful in predicting whether and how much a patient will improve, but care must be taken in correlating MRI pattern with clinical outcome.

Treatment

Compression fractures heal quickly with little tendency to further progression. Thus, for the mild injury, symptomatic treatment is sufficient with a short period of bed rest or immobilization with a cast or a corset [40]. Many children can be treated at home or require only a short period in hospital. In reports comparing casts to bed rest, the specific treatment did not affect the outcome, and the children were generally asymptomatic in 1–2 weeks [13, 26, 31]. Posterior tenderness in the area of the fracture occasionally persists but does not pose a serious problem [26]. If the endplate is fractured and the disc herniates into the vertebral body, symptoms may persist but can be expected to resolve with symptomatic treatment. However, the kyphotic deformity due to damaged vertebral endplates may not resolve without specific management (see section "Lumbar and Dorsolumbar Scheuermann's Disease"). Thoracic and lumbar vertebral fractures in late adolescence with no or minor neurological deficits have predominantly favorable long-term outcome, even if no remodeling capacity of the fractured vertebral body remains [72]. Sagittal spinal canal width and kyphosis increased in absolute values from baseline to follow-up at all levels, while the disc heights, the degrees of scoliosis, the degree of anterior, posterior, and lateral displacements were unchanged. Prevalence of back pain up to 47 years after vertebral fracture was no higher than expected in a general population [72].

Children who sustain an unstable injury, such as a vertebral subluxation or a fracture dislocation, should undergo reduction in the same manner as an adult with a similar injury [13, 23, 31, 73, 74]. Early surgical treatment, instrumentation, and fusion are mandatory for unstable fractures and injuries associated with spinal cord lesions. In children, a traumatic spinal cord lesion may develop a deformity that is mainly scoliotic, kyphotic, or lordotic in 90% of cases [40]. The child should be nursed on a turning frame or with complete bed rest and logrolling until the acute symptoms subside. The dislocation should be reduced promptly in the neurologically injured child, particularly those with a low

lesion that involves the conus medullaris and nerve roots. Risk of neurological injury increases with canal narrowing, at T1–T12 (35%), L1 (45%), and L2 and below (55%) [71]. The average canal compromise in six adolescents with burst fractures was 55% at the time of injury but only one had an incomplete neurological deficit [75]. Thomas et al. [41] investigated multi-level burst fractures and found neurological deficits in 80% (four of five) patients, which is substantially greater than the 65% reported in single-level burst fractures. Children with burst fractures that result in spinal canal narrowing (greater than 25%) and kyphosis are at increased risk of further canal compromise and should be considered for early correction and decompression [23, 40]. Lalonde et al. [75] found that (a) children who sustain burst fractures tend to develop mild progressive angular deformity at the site of the fracture, (b) operative stabilization prevented further kyphotic deformity as well as decreasing the length of hospitalization without contributing to further cord compromise, and (c) nonoperative treatment of burst fracture was a viable option in neurologically intact children, but progressive angular deformity occurred during the first year after the fracture. In the long term, those who were corrected lost an additional 11% of kyphosis and 12% of anterior vertebral compression. In the nonoperative group, an average of 33% worsened and anterior vertebral compression worsened on average 8%. They concluded that growth proceeded normally in the posterior column and was relatively absent anteriorly. As in the adult, spinal instrumentation is helpful in reducing the deformity and stabilizing the fracture site [11, 12, 76, 77]. Open reduction must be accompanied by a posterior spinal fusion at least one level above and below the fracture site. Spontaneous interbody fusion seldom occurs and should not be depended on to provide long-term stability [13, 31]. Injuries that would be classified as stable in the adult may spontaneously progress in the child. This is common when there has been severe crushing of the vertebral body and endplate (burst fracture) and disruption of the posterior support ligaments or laminectomy [13]. McPhee [13] suggests that this may represent a Salter type IV injury to the vertebral epiphysis, with a growth arrest leading to progressive deformity. Early recognition, reduction, and surgical stabilization will prevent late deformity [13]. In the older child, Lancourt et al. [12] have suggested extending the fusion to include the sacrum as a guard against the late onset of scoliosis. Thomas et al. [41] conclude that multiple burst fractures should be treated individually based on their clinical and radiographic characteristics. Early reduction of the deformity and surgical stabilization will prevent the problems of progressive kyphosis or late neurological injury [73–75].

Laminectomy is seldom helpful, particularly in the child without bony injury [11, 13, 17, 40, 64, 73, 77, 78]. The indications for immediate surgical decompression are the same as those in the adult: (i) an open wound (ii) progressive neurological deficit in an incomplete injury, and (iii) reduction of an unstable fracture dislocation [17, 79]. Removal of the posterior elements frequently accentuates the already unstable condition and may lead to progressive deformity [14]. Laminectomy is not a cause of scoliosis, but many children develop significant kyphosis following the procedure, which is difficult to manage [12, 14, 27, 64, 77]. It would seem advisable that, if a laminectomy is necessary, it should be accompanied by a short segment fusion. Parisini et al. [40] reported on some patients who developed significant kyphoscoliosis at follow-up. The residual deformity involved more segments above and below the level of the lesion. All the patients who progressed had inadequate instrumentation. Distraction-type instrumentation, such as the Harrington rod, was unable to stabilize the lesion.

Neurological Injury

The most devastating problem for the child with a thoracolumbar spine injury is paraplegia, which can be associated with all the problems seen in the adult: increased susceptibility to long bone fractures, hip dislocation, pressure sores, joint contractures, and genitourinary complications [4, 79, 80]. In addition, the child can be expected to develop progressive spinal deformity (scoliosis, kyphosis, and lordosis) that will significantly complicate management [11, 40, 64, 79, 81]. For many, the original injury is often overshadowed by the severity of these late spinal deformities [4]. Scoliosis seriously erodes the child's ability to sit easily, and in the young child, pelvic obliquity leads to subluxation of the hip and ischial pressure sores [12, 82]. Kilfoyle et al.

[82] noted in 1965 that "Surgical intervention is now considered an expression of conservatism." Inexplicably, this recommendation continues to be rediscovered with each subsequent article on the problem of progressive scoliosis in the immature paraplegic and quadriplegic.

In immature children, usually girls under 12 years and boys under 14 years, the incidence of progressive spine deformity following traumatic paraplegia is 86–100% [4, 7, 11, 12, 80] (Fig. 6.12). The onset of curvature has been reported as early as 3 years of age [15]. The fracture seldom determines the direction of the spinal curvature, rather the majority develop a long paralytic thoracolumbar curve believed to be due to the influence of gravity and uneven forces of spasticity [12, 82]. Similarly, on the lateral radiograph the predominant finding (57%) is a reversal of the normal lumbar lordosis with the development of a long thoracolumbar kyphosis, with its apex at the dorsolumbar junction [11, 12]. Progressive lumbar lordosis is less common (18%) and usually associated with hip flexion contractures, particularly in the ambulatory patient [11, 12, 83]. Progression of the spinal curvature is directly related to the age of the child, spasticity, and the level of the lesion [11, 12]. Children with more proximal injuries are more likely to have a progressive deformity than those injured at or below the level of the conus medullaris [4, 79, 83].

In adolescents who are nearly skeletally mature at the time of injury, spinal deformity is more often due to a fracture dislocation [11]. Progressive kyphosis and pain at the fracture site are common (42%), particularly in those who underwent laminectomy [11, 64, 81, 82].

If the kyphotic deformity is progressive, long-term neurological sequelae may develop with further loss of function

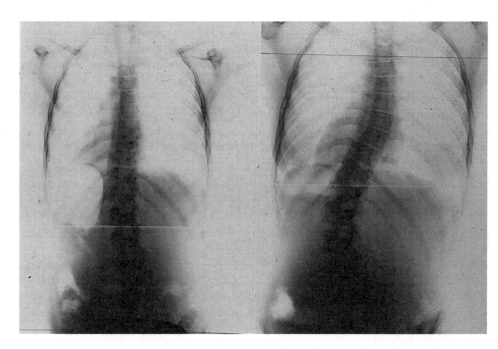

Fig. 6.12 Radiograph of a 9-year-old girl who sustained multiple trauma in a motor vehicle accident. There was no vertebral fracture identified but she had a complete transverse myelitis at T10, believed to be due to vascular injury. (**a**) AP view at 11 years demonstrates a mild collapsing-type curvature. (**b**) At 14 years the curve has increased to 50° despite vigorous management with an underarm orthosis and excellent compliance by the patient. Surgical stabilization and correction of the spine are required to prevent further deformity. From: Rockwood CA, Wilkin KE, Beaty JH, eds. Fractures in Children, Volume 3, 4th Edition, Philadelphia: Lippincott-Raven, 1996. Used with permission

from tenting of the spinal cord over the kyphus. Thus, early surgical stabilization should be considered [11].

Treatment of scoliosis should be initiated soon after the injury, prior to developing a severe curve. The Milwaukee brace has not been effective in controlling a collapsing paralytic curve; however, a total contact underarm plastic orthosis (TLSO) has been helpful [79]. Treatment recommendations are similar to those for idiopathic scoliosis. Curves under 40–45° may be controlled by bracing, or at least surgery can be delayed until the child is of optimum age [12, 19, 81]. Once the curve exceeds 45–50°, surgical stabilization should proceed promptly [11, 79, 81]. In Mayfield's series, 68% required surgical correction [11]. It is helpful if the sacrum is not included in the fusion, as this significantly increases the incidence of pseudoarthrosis.

Post-traumatic Syrinx

With the more frequent use of MRI, the relatively rare problem of post-traumatic syringomyelia is being discovered with greater frequency [66]. Symptoms can develop as late as 17 years after injury (average 4.5 years) [84, 85]. Pain is the initial symptom in over half, followed by progressive neurological deterioration, sweating below the original lesion, and loss of motor function and deep tendon reflexes are indications of a progressive syrinx [85]. MRI is excellent in identifying the lesion and Betz advocates an initial baseline MRI in these children to facilitate later detection [66, 84].

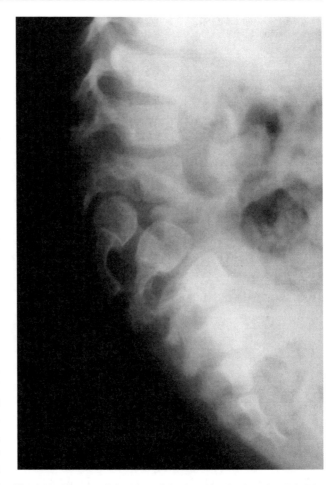

Fig. 6.13 Fracture dislocation of the dorsal lumbar junction (L2–L3), secondary to child abuse. This injury is believed to be secondary to spanking with resultant partial paraplegia

Differential Diagnosis

Child Abuse

Vertebral injuries due to child abuse are less common than those of the extremities [15, 21]. The injuries are usually due to hyperflexion and may be simple compression of the vertebral bodies, avulsion of the secondary center of ossification of the spinous process, less frequently herniation of the nucleus pulposus into the vertebral body, and rarely a fracture dislocation and kyphosis due to severe disruption [21, 86–89] (Fig. 6.13). A striking example is the report of subluxation of T12 on L1 with complete paraplegia from spanking [90]. A thoracolumbar fracture dislocation or listhesis injury resulting from abuse can be misinterpreted as an infectious process or congenital. Levin et al. [20] reported that additional skeletal findings of abuse, while present in some cases, were not universal. There are no radiological vertebral changes specific for battering. Similarly, the classic epiphyseal and metaphyseal fractures of the long bones

associated with battering are present in only 15% of all abused children [89]. Clinically, a high index of suspicion is more important than a specific radiographic finding (see Chapter 5 of Children's Upper and Lower Limb Fractures).

Carrion et al. [91] noted that certain dorsolumbar junction injuries in the young child may be from spanking, representing child abuse, and are analogous to a Salter–Harris type I fracture in a long bone. The fracture is usually through the vertebral body at T12 along the neural central synchondrosis across the inferior endplate and intervertebral disc, exiting anteriorly in the superior (or inferior) endplate of L1 [91] and may slide forward [20].

Systemic Diseases

Spontaneous collapse of a single vertebra should alert one to the possibility of eosinophilic granuloma of the spine. Most of the children are between 2 and 5 years old [43]. Usually there is a complete collapse of the body (vertebra plana), and seldom does one see the lytic appearance that is

Fig. 6.14 (**a**) An 8-year-old with spontaneous onset of vertebral pain in the thoracic spine. The diagnosis was not confirmed by biopsy, as the clinical presentation was typical of vertebral eosinophilic granuloma. She was treated symptomatically in a TLSO with complete recovery and about 40% reconstitution. No further signs of histocytosis X were found. (**b**) A 7-year-old child demonstrating a rare herniation of the eosinophilic granuloma into the thoracic spinal column. The child presented with clonus and hyperreflexia. Anterior excision confirmed the eosinophilic granuloma. The lesion was bone grafted and healed without incident

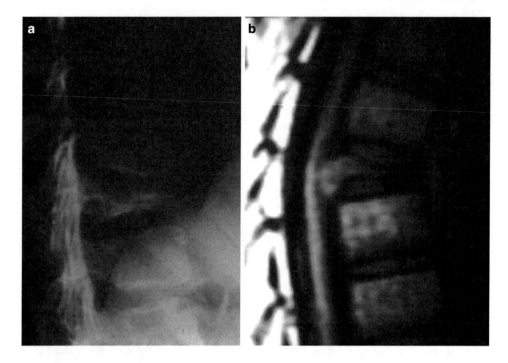

typical of skeletal involvement in other areas (Fig. 6.14). The intervertebral disc is not affected and its thickness is retained. An adjacent soft tissue mass is uncommon, and if present, it suggests an infectious process such as tuberculosis. Several vertebral bodies may be involved, and as many as 11 have been reported [92]. The prognosis is excellent with some growth in height of the vertebral body and little residual deformity. However, complete restitution seldom occurs. We have seen Ewing's sarcoma present as vertebra plana, usually with a soft tissue mass.

Multiple vertebral collapse is commonly seen in Gaucher's disease, mucopolysaccharidoses, lymphoma (Fig. 6.15), and neuroblastoma [93, 94]. The abnormal cells displace normal bone; the vertebra becomes structurally weak and collapses with minor trauma. Usually the children have visceral as well as skeletal involvement at other sites. A bone scan should be obtained to identify other sites. Typical symptoms are persistent back pain localized to the region of the collapse. Neurological complications are rare.

In Gaucher's disease[93], the bone-forming elements are replaced by an infiltrate of carosen-containing reticulum cells. This can usually be confirmed by aspiration of the marrow and finding the atypical cells [93]. One or more vertebrae may collapse, but a gibbus is rare [93] (Fig. 6.16). Schmorl's node formation may occur.

The mucopolysaccharides, chondrodystrophies, and lipidoses are similar to Gaucher's, with cellular storage of an abnormal metabolite and structural weakness. Vertebral changes are typically first noted at the dorsolumbar junction, with anterior herniation of the nucleus pulposus, and radiologically appear as a "beaking" of the vertebral body

(Fig. 6.17). Depending on the severity of the disease, the process may involve the entire spine [23].

Vertebral compression fractures can be seen in a significant number of chronically ill children and are poorly predicted by single bone mineral density (BMD) measurements and clinical history [95]. Seventy-eight percent had a history of treatment with steroids for a median duration of 13 months. Weight and BMD were significantly higher in the group with significant spinal changes. This difference was independent of the cumulative steroid dose, suggesting that increased body weight may predispose these patients to compression fractures [95].

Compression fractures are common in osteogenesis imperfecta (Fig. 6.18) and may develop serially, similar to the storage diseases. However, the children may have typical stigmata such as blue sclerae, fragility of the long bones, and deformity of the extremities (see Chapter 6 of General Principles of Children's Orthopaedic Disease). Progressive spinal deformity, scoliosis, and kyphosis are common in the severely involved children. Certain conditions are associated with systemic osteoporosis and can lead to compression fractures with kyphosis such as cystic fibrosis or as a consequence of treatment, such as steroid-induced osteoporosis in children with severe juvenile idiopathic arthritis [96, 97] (see Chapter 12 of General Principles of Children's Orthopaedic Disease).

Assessment of vertebral morphology is recommended as an additional tool in the diagnostic workup of paediatric osteoporosis [95]. Compression fractures occur with idiopathic juvenile osteoporosis, an unusual acquired systemic condition characterized by profound osteoporosis in an

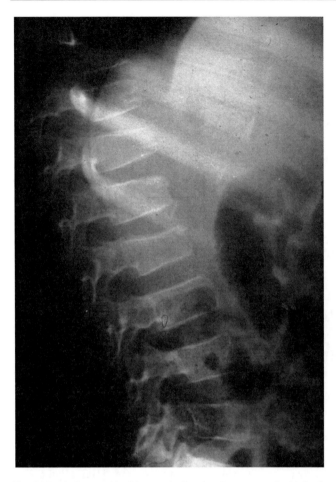

Fig. 6.15 A 6-year-old with acute leukemia who presented with back pain and multiple compression fractures of the lumbar spine. This was a spontaneous onset with no history of trauma initially believed to represent child abuse until leukemia was diagnosed

otherwise normal prepubertal child, typically between age 8 and 15 years [98] (see Chapter 6 of General Principles of Children's Orthopaedic Disease). Initial complaints are usually related to the spine and the tibia and if the condition is recognized, early treatment with a spine brace will improve appearance and reduce the degree of kyphosis and residual deformity [98].

Lumbar and Dorsolumbar Scheuermann's Disease

Scheuermann's disease is a common cause of thoracic kyphosis. The condition is seldom painful. Typically children present with concerns related to the appearance of the deformity and are found to have the characteristic vertebral changes. Sorenson's radiographic criteria, which include three or more adjacent vertebrae wedged greater than 50%, have been generally accepted to confirm the diagnosis [47,

99, 100]. Endplate irregularity, Schmorl's node formation, and narrowing of the disc space are commonly seen but are not in themselves diagnostic [101]. Lumbar or dorsolumbar osteochondritis is less common but more often accompanied by pain [102, 103]. Several authors, including Scheuermann [104], suggest that the lumbar vertebral changes are the result of trauma [102–104]. By contrast, typical thoracic Scheuermann's disease is limited to the thoracic vertebrae, spontaneous in onset, and due to hereditary influences [100]. Clinically, lumbar or dorsolumbar Scheuermann's disease primarily affects adolescents (13–17 years) and is accompanied by a period of moderately severe pain with activity [100]. Usually the children have a history of previous acute strain or injury [102, 103, 105]. The lumbar vertebral changes are often associated with hard physical labor before the age of 16, suggesting that the maturing endplate and vertebral body are more vulnerable to increased mechanical strain during this period of rapid growth [102, 103]. Hafner [106] coined the term apprentice kyphosis, or kyphosis muscularis, and he found that it occurred more commonly in boys (2:1) between the ages of 15 and 17 during the growth spurt [106]. Micheli found similar lumbar changes to be common in young athletes and suggested that the etiology was a localized stress injury to the vertebral growth plates [107].

The apophyseal bony centers appear first in the lower thoracic region at approximately 9 years of age and fuse with the vertebral body between the age of 17 and 22 years. The ring is thinner in the middle than in the periphery. In the laboratory, Jayson et al. [108] found that mechanically increasing the pressure in the intervertebral disc will force it through the center of the endplate and into the cancellous bone of the vertebral body (Fig. 6.19). The mechanism is analogous to the production of Schmorl's nodes and is accompanied by narrowing of the disc space [108, 109]. Similarly, metabolic and neoplastic diseases that lead to structural weakening of the bone are often associated with Schmorl's node formation [109]. Alexander [110] found that marginal Schmorl's nodes are more often associated with trauma and central nodes are more frequent and consistent with thoracic Scheuermann's disease [74]. Heavy lifting, especially when seated and bending forward, increases the intranuclear pressures to the lower end of the range necessary in experimental models to achieve fracture through the normal vertebral endplate [108] (Fig. 6.20). Micheli [107] noted that the flexion–extension motion of the spine seen in rowers, weight lifters, and gymnasts can achieve these same forces (Fig. 6.21).

In an acute traumatic disc herniation, the disc space is narrowed and the anterior angle of the inferior vertebra slightly flattened, giving an anterior wedged appearance. The Schmorl's node itself may not be visible on plain films and seen only on laminograms or CT reconstruction (Fig. 6.19). After 2–3 months, the radiolucent defect is clearly visible in

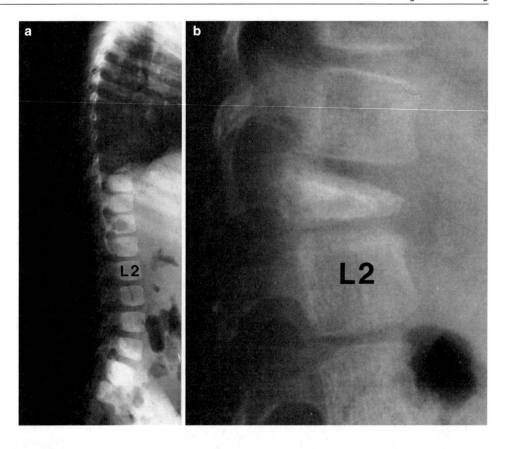

Fig. 6.16 Gaucher's disease. The illness is progressive with increased storage of the abnormal metabolite and structural weakening of the vertebral elements. (**a**) Normal appearance of the thoracolumbar spine at age 5 years. (**b**) At age 8 years, a spontaneous compression fracture of L1 has occurred. The patient sustained many similar fractures until her death 3 years later. From: Rockwood CA, Wilkin KE, Beaty JH, eds. Fractures in Children, Volume 3, 4th Edition, Philadelphia: Lippincott-Raven, 1996. Used with permission

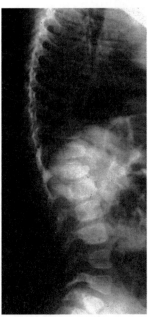

Fig. 6.17 Radiograph of a 13-month-old infant evaluated for delay in motor milestones and subluxation of the hips. Lateral view of the spine demonstrates a beaking of L2 vertebral body. This finding is compatible with a storage disease such as mucopolysaccharidosis, or mucolipidosis, or hypothyroidism. Further clinical and laboratory investigations are indicated. In this child, laboratory studies have confirmed the diagnosis of Hurler's syndrome

the inferior vertebra as the localization has been enhanced by reactive sclerosis in the adjacent bone [105] (Fig. 6.22). There is also buttressing occurring as a thin rim of periosteal new bone under the anterior longitudinal ligament. In some children the disc material may pass peripherally, usually anterior, and submarginally beneath the apophyseal ring [102, 103, 111] (Fig. 6.22). Radiologically, this appears as a separation of the triangular bone fragment from the vertebral body that represents the ring apophysis [111]. Less commonly, posterior separation may occur with narrowing of the spinal canal (see section "Slipped Vertebral Apophysis"). The defect may heal with growth, but typically the apophysis remains separate from the vertebral body, the so-called limbus vertebra [111]. The condition can be encountered at any site, but occurs most often at the dorsolumbar junction, and at more than one level [103, 106, 107].

Clinical symptoms of back pain may extend over 2–6 months, are increased by activity and forward flexion, and are relieved by rest [102, 103].

Conservative treatment such as enforced rest or bracing is usually sufficient. Occasionally, the patient will require bed rest or plaster immobilization. There are no reports of children who have required surgical intervention for the control of symptoms and only a few have required correction for deformity. The vertebral changes improve slowly during

Fig. 6.18 Osteogenesis imperfecta. (**a**) Lateral radiograph of the spine at age 4 years with compression fractures of the lumbar vertebrae. (**b**) At age 7 years, compression fractures of every vertebra, with extreme narrowing of the vertebral body and apparent increase of the intervertebral spaces representing the discs that have retained their normal elasticity. From: Rockwood CA, Wilkin KE, Beaty JH, eds. Fractures in Children, Volume 3, 4th Edition, Philadelphia: Lippincott-Raven, 1996. Used with permission

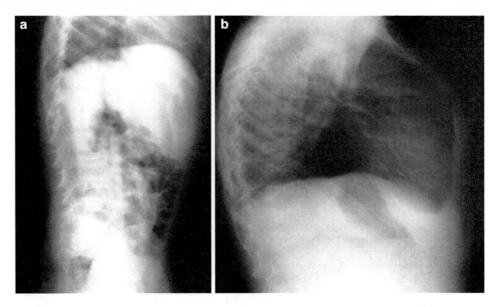

Fig. 6.19 Radiographs of a 15-year-old boy with persistent back pain in the mid-lumbar region following a weight-lifting program. (**a**) Routine lateral view suggests mild endplate changes. (**b**) Laminagraphic view demonstrates Schmorl's node formation and endplate irregularity of T11. Subtle changes in routine films may belie significant endplate changes or disc protrusion into the vertebral body

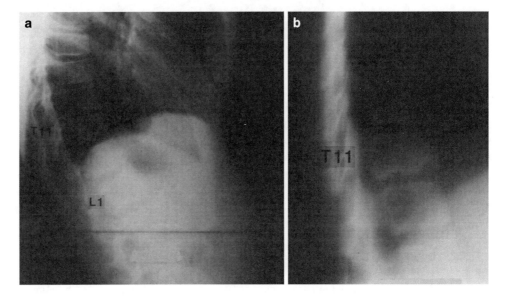

growth. Schmorl's node formation and disc space narrowing generally persist [105]. Similarly, the separate apophyseal fragment at the anterior margin of the vertebral body seldom heals (Fig. 6.17).

Progressive kyphosis may ensue due to two mechanisms: (i) the anterior deformation of the vertebral bodies from the original injury and (ii) the increased pressure on the anterior margin, which may lead to cessation of growth in that region (Fig. 6.23). However, the kyphosis is generally not severe and seldom requires any treatment. If the deformity is significant and the child is skeletally immature, a Milwaukee brace is recommended.

Traumatic Spondylolysis

Spondylolysis at L5 to S1 is often referred to as a congenital anomaly of the spine, yet there is no supporting embryological or anatomical evidence for this assumption. Despite an anatomical incidence of 5% in the general population, only one infant has been discovered to have the pars interarticularis defect [112–114]. Spondylolysis in children occurs after walking age but rarely before 5 years of age and more commonly at 7 or 8 years, suggesting that trauma is an important etiological factor [112, 115]. However, Rowe

Fig. 6.20 A 14-year-old male with back pain following repetitive injury to the lumbar spine by lifting weights. (**a**) Lumbar spine radiograph demonstrates a Schmorl's node on the cephalad portion of the L3 vertebra and on the caudal portion of the L2 vertebra. (**b**) MRI of the same vertebrae demonstrating extensive reaction to the Schmorl's node more acute in the vertebral body of L4 and more chronic in L2

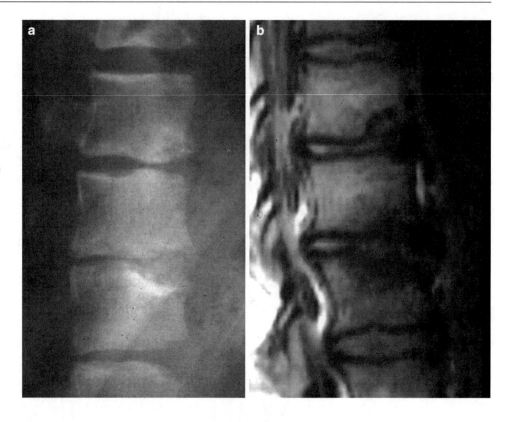

[112] was unable to produce the typical pars interarticularis lesion in infant cadavers despite vigorous flexion and extension. Hitchcock [116] could produce spondylolysis only by forced hyperflexion, and laboratory tests indicate that a high degree of force is required. A history of minor but seldom severe trauma is common (50% of males and 25% of females) and is often related to the onset of symptoms which coincide closely with the adolescent growth spurt [117–120].

There is substantial documentation that spondylolysis represents a "stress" or fatigue fracture of the pars interarticularis [121]. It is postulated that lumbar lordosis is accentuated by the normal hip flexion contractures of childhood. This posture focuses the force of weight bearing on the pars interarticularis, leading to gradual disruptions. Anatomical studies suggest that shear stresses are greater on the pars interarticularis when the spine is extended [121]. In children and adolescents the pars interarticularis is thin, the neural arch has not reached its maximum strength, and the intervertebral disc is less resistant to shear [121]. A fatigue fracture can occur at physiological loads during cyclic flexion–extension of the lumbar spine [121] (Fig. 6.24). Jackson noted spondylolysis to be four times more common (11%) in female gymnasts than expected. Some initially had normal roentgenograms and later developed spondylolysis [122] (Fig. 6.25).

An increased incidence of traumatic spondylolysis (32–50%) has been noted in teenagers with dorsolumbar Scheuermann's disease, a condition believed to be caused by excessive and repetitive mechanical loading of the immature spine [103, 123]. Similarly, dorsolumbar kyphosis is often associated with a compensatory increase in lumbar lordosis [123]. An increased incidence has been noted in those performing heavy physical work such as weight lifters, lumbermen, and football linemen [124].

Several findings favor a congenital origin. A high rate of incidence among family members and certain ethnic groups has been reported by numerous authors: 27–69% in near relatives versus an expected frequency of 4–8% in the general population [125]. There is racial and sex difference, with the lowest incidence in black females and the highest (6.4%) in white males [112]. People with spondylolysis have an increased incidence of sacral spina bifida (28–42%) and a congenital lack of development of the proximal sacrum and superior sacral facets [125].

Thus, there is supporting data in favor of both developmental and congenital origins for spondylolysis. Congenital deficiency of the sacrum and lack of integrity of the posterior structures, on a genetic basis, may predispose a person to spondylolysis. Developmental factors such as trauma, posture, or certain repetitive activities may lead to a stress fracture of the pars interarticularis.

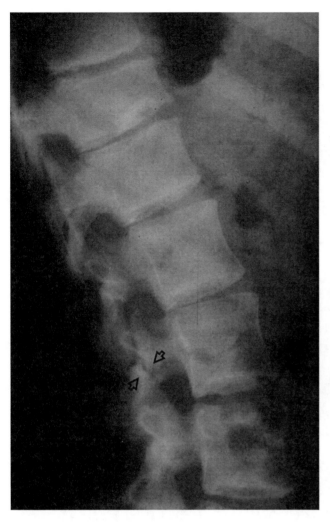

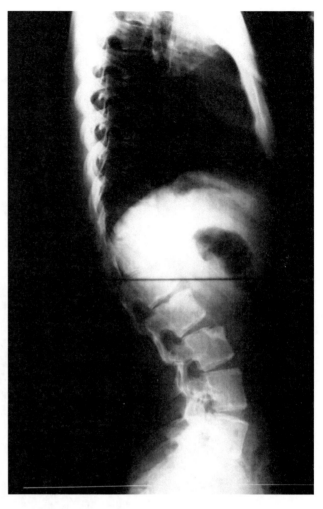

Fig. 6.21 Radiograph of a 13-year-old male who sustained vertebral endplate changes at several levels while playing football. Note the associated spondylolysis (*arrows*). The patient's persistent discomfort responded satisfactorily to bracing

Fig. 6.23 Lumbar Scheuermann's disease in a 16-year-old male who sustained anterior compression and kyphosis at the dorsolumbar junction. He had persistent discomfort over several months that responded to bracing. Note several vertebrae have Schmorl's node formation and the kyphosis is localized at the dorsolumbar junction with increased lumbar lordosis

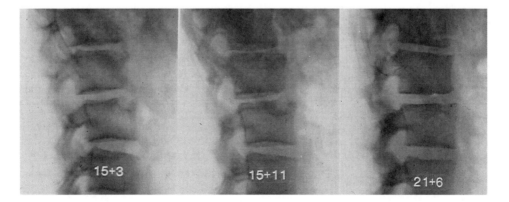

Fig. 6.22 Acute herniated Schmorl's node. (**a**) Radiographs of a 15-year-old weight lifter with back pain and Schmorl's nodes at L2, L3, and L4. (**b**) Eight months later, there has been continued growth of the vertebrae without progressive deformity. (**c**) At 22 years of age the sites of the Schmorl's nodes are still seen, although they appear smaller. The minimal wedging at L2 has not changed in the preceding 6 years. From: Rockwood CA, Wilkin KE, Beaty JH, eds. Fractures in Children, Volume 3, 4th Edition, Philadelphia: Lippincott-Raven, 1996. Used with permission

Fig. 6.24 A 10-year old with spondylolysis. (**a**) Extension and (**b**) flexion views. Note the change in the gap and the flexibility of the disc. The child was asymptomatic. He was not expected to develop symptoms until he is closer to his teenage years, if at all

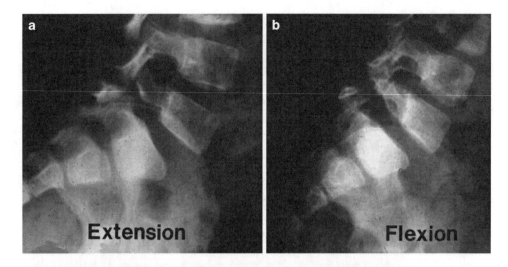

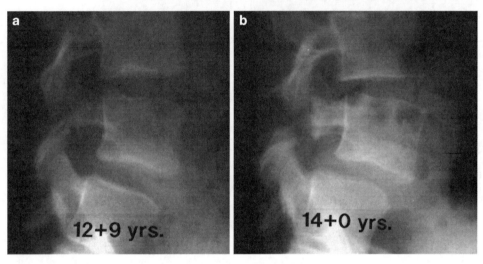

Fig. 6.25 (**a**) Radiograph of a 12-year- and 10-month-old male with normal appearance of the lumbosacral junction. (**b**) The same patient at age 14 years. Spondylolysis and grade I spondylolisthesis have developed in the interim with symptoms referable to the low back.

Spondylolysis in children occurs after walking age, but rarely before 5 years, and more commonly at 7 or 8 years. Onset of symptoms coincides closely with the adolescent growth spurt

Symptoms and Signs

Spondylolysis commonly occurs in late childhood or early adolescence; however, symptoms are relatively uncommon in children and often not sufficiently severe to require medical attention during the teenage years [126, 127]. In a prospective longitudinal study, only 13% of children known to have spondylolysis developed symptoms before 18 years of age [126]. For the occasional child who may develop symptoms, the onset usually coincides with the adolescent growth spurt [117].

Although pain is the predominant complaint in adults, a significant number of children do not have pain and are referred for a postural deformity or abnormality of gait due to hamstring tightness. If the child does complain of pain,

the pain is generally localized to the low back and, to a lesser extent, to the posterior buttocks and thighs [117, 119]. Symptoms are usually related to strenuous exercise, particularly repetitive flexion–extension of the spine common as in rowing, diving, serving in tennis, and gymnastics and are decreased by rest or limitation of activity [107, 117, 121, 122].

Children, unlike adults, seldom have objective signs of nerve root compression, such as motor weakness, reflex change, or sensory deficit [120]. However, examination should include a careful search for sacral anesthesia and bladder dysfunction. Similarly, children with spondylolysis rarely have myelographic evidence of disc protrusion, and in those explored for herniation, none were found [117, 120].

Hamstring tightness (so-called spasm) is commonly found in 80% of symptomatic patients and thought by some to be

Fig. 6.26 (a) Pars interarticularis defect, spondylolysis, as seen on oblique radiograph view (*arrow*), typically found with the isthmic type of spondylolisthesis. (**b**) Similar oblique view of a patient with dysplastic (congenital) spondylolisthesis, demonstrating elongation and attenuation of the pars interarticularis, perhaps a prespondylolytic defect, and possibly representing a "stress" or fatigue fracture of the pars interarticularis. From: Rockwood CA, Wilkin KE, Beaty JH, eds. Fractures in Children, Volume 3, 4th Edition, Philadelphia: Lippincott-Raven, 1996. Used with permission

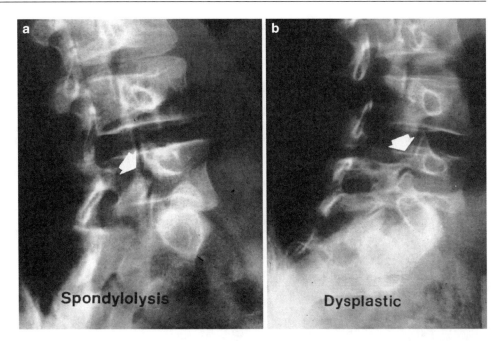

a sign of nerve root irritation but there is no evidence to support this contention [115, 120]. Severe hamstring tightness may be found in patients with spondylolysis or with all grades of spondylolisthesis but is seldom accompanied by neurological signs [115, 117, 119]. Physical examination may demonstrate some tenderness on palpation of the lower back. There may be some splinting, guarding, and restriction of side-to-side motion particularly if the condition is of acute onset. If tightness of the hamstrings is present, there will be marked restriction of forward flexion at the hips.

Imaging Features

Spondylolysis refers to the radiolucent defect in the pars interarticularis (Fig. 6.21). If the defect is large, it can be seen on nearly all radiographs of the lumbar spine. If unilateral, as occurs in 20% of patients, or not accompanied by spondylolisthesis, it can be a very subtle finding requiring special techniques such as oblique views of the lumbar spine [128] (Fig. 6.26). Particularly, in young, symptomatic patients, if oblique views are not obtained, the diagnosis can be missed in up to 20%. The "Scotty dog" of Lachapelle with the defect appearing at the neck is a helpful visual aid to those inexperienced with oblique radiographs (Fig. 6.27). In an acute injury, the gap is narrow with irregular edges, whereas in the long-standing lesion, the edges are smooth and rounded, suggesting a pseudarthrosis (Fig. 6.26). The width of the gap depends on the amount of bone resorption following the fracture and the degree of spondylolisthesis.

Less commonly, children may have poorly developed posterior structures, referred to by Wiltse et al. [114] as the dysplastic (type I), and due to the anomalous development, the posterior facets appear to subluxate on the sacral facets. This is a common finding in children who are symptomatic (26–35%) [124]. In children with the dysplastic type, rather than a gap or a defect in the pars interarticularis, the facets appear to subluxate on the radiograph and the pars interarticularis may become attenuated, the "greyhound" sign of Hensinger [117] (Fig. 6.26), and later a defect may appear in the center. Wiltse et al. [114] suggest that they are different manifestations of the same disease process, as he and Wynne-Davies and Scott [125] have found both lesions present in family members, suggesting that the spondylolytic type represents an acute stress fracture of the pars interarticularis and the dysplastic or elongated type represents a chronic stress reaction with gradual attenuation of the pars.

Deficiency of the posterior elements is a common occurrence in spondylolysis. Easily observable defects, such as dysraphic or malformed laminae, have been found in 32–94% of these patients, and if discovered on routine lumbosacral views, a more detailed radiographic investigation should be performed [125]. CT is rarely indicated in acute fracture of the pars interarticularis, as a combination of bone scan and oblique films will more reliably detect the lesion [129]. Similarly, spondylolysis at other levels, such as L4 or L3, is more difficult to diagnose with CT because the plane of scanning is parallel to the fracture [129]. MRI should be considered if the patient's symptoms or neurological signs do not resolve with bed rest. Similarly, bladder and bowel dysfunction or perineal hypesthesia justify further investigation.

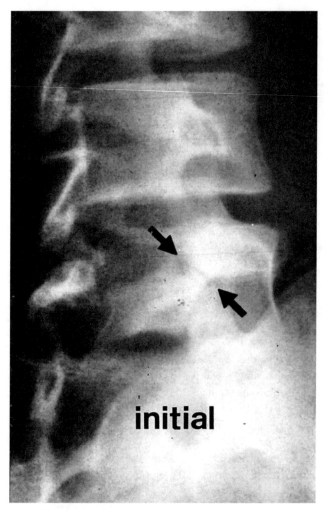

Fig. 6.27 Radiograph of a 13-year-old boy who felt a "snap" in the low back during a swimming racing turn. Radiograph demonstrates spondylolysis of the pars interarticularis (*arrows*). The narrow, irregular appearance suggests recent injury. From: Rockwood CA, Wilkin KE, Beaty JH, eds. Fractures in Children, Volume 3, 4th Edition, Philadelphia: Lippincott-Raven, 1996. Used with permission

Sherman and associates [118] described the unusual appearance of reactive sclerosis and hypertrophy of the pedicle and lamina and contralateral spondylolysis in the same vertebral segment (Fig. 6.28). They suggest that this represents a physiological response to stress, the result of repeated trauma in the presence of an unstable neural arch that will respond to conservative measures and symptomatic treatment [118]. Radiologically, this may be confused with the reactive sclerosis associated with an osteoid osteoma. This is important as excision of a sclerotic pedicle associated with a contralateral spondylolysis may increase instability. The presence of a nidus on the CT scan should confirm the diagnosis of an osteoid osteoma. A bone scan will not be helpful in differentiating between the two, since both will exhibit increased isotope uptake.

Bone Scans

Children who are suspected clinically but cannot be confirmed radiologically, particularly those in the stress reaction (prespondylolytic) stage prior to fracture, may be detected by radioactive bone scan [107, 130]. Those with small, partial, or unilateral fractures can be overlooked on plain radiographs, but bone scan will always demonstrate areas of increased bone turnover, due to the healing fracture. Positive bone scans are associated with a short clinical history and may demonstrate increased uptake in those with only 5–7 days of symptoms [130, 131]. Later the bone scan is helpful to distinguish between those with an established nonunion and those in whom healing is still progressing and may benefit from immobilization [121, 131]. The bone scan is not recommended in those whose symptoms are of more than 1 year duration or for those who do not have symptoms [131]. The bone scan is particularly helpful for those whose activities are particularly associated with spondylolysis, such as gymnasts [122]. Early detection of the stress reaction may lead to appropriate treatment and shorten the recovery period.

Fig. 6.28 Radiographs of a 15-year-old boy with low back pain. Anterior and posterior (**a**) and oblique (**b** and **c**) views demonstrate reactive sclerosis and hypertrophy of one pedicle and lamina (*arrow*), and a contralateral spondylolysis of the same vertebral segment. The oblique view (**b**) demonstrates the reactive sclerosis. Radiologically, this may be confused with an osteoid osteoma

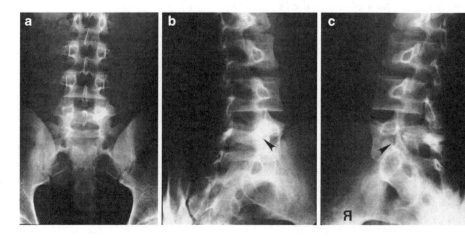

Similarly, the bone scan can be used to assess recovery and prior to the athlete returning to competitions [122]. The bone scan is not indicated once the lesion has become established, unless one suspects bone tumor such as osteoid osteoma, infection, or malignancy.

Treatment

Several authors have reported children and young adults who have been able to heal the spondylolytic defect with a cast or a brace (TLSO) [107, 131]. Typically, the children have an acute onset of symptoms and the episode of injury can be clearly documented. Unfortunately, not all heal with immobilization. However, immobilization should be considered if the injury can be documented to be of recent origin. A bone scan may be helpful to indicate a continuing process versus one of long duration [121].

Although healing is unlikely, in children and teenagers whom the spondylolysis is of long duration, can be expected to respond clinically to simple conservative measures [127]. Restriction of vigorous activities and back and abdominal strengthening exercises are usually successful in controlling those with mild back ache and hamstring tightness [127]. Patients with more severe or persistent complaints may require bed rest, immobilization in a cast or a brace, and non-narcotic analgesics. Hamstring tightness is an excellent clinical guide to the success or the failure of the treatment program. The majority of affected children have excellent relief of symptoms or only minimal discomfort on long-term follow-up [120].

Any child or adolescent with symptoms due to spondylolysis, especially those under 10 years of age, should be followed closely for progression to spondylolisthesis [127]. We do not advise those with asymptomatic spondylolysis or those with minimal symptoms to restrict their activities. About 7.2% of asymptomatic young men aged 18–30 years have a pars defect, and relatively few have persistent symptoms. Thus, limitation of activity in a growing child would not seem justified [107, 127].

It must be emphasized that it is uncommon for spondylolysis to be symptomatic in adolescence, and one should be particularly wary of the child whose symptoms do not respond to bed rest or who has objective neurological findings. In this situation, MRI and electromyographic investigation should be considered.

A small percentage of young people with spondylolysis do not respond to conservative measures or are unwilling to curtail their activities and may require surgical stabilization. If surgery for spondylolysis is found necessary, a lateral column fusion from L5 to S1 employing iliac bone

is usually sufficient. In those who also have a spondylolisthesis of grade III or greater, the fusion is usually extended to L4 [127]. Nachemson [132] reported solid healing of the defect using a bone graft coupled with an intertransverse process fusion. In those patients in whom the defect is small (6–7 mm) and the degree of spondylolisthesis is slight, a variety of techniques have been described to reduce the defect directly. These include wiring of the transverse process or screw placement across the pars with bone grafting [133–136]. These procedures are usually recommended for the older teenager and young adult less than 30 years of age with a minimal degree of displacement and degenerative change [135]. The best candidates are those with defects between L1 and L4 [133–136]. This is an attractive alternative to the traditional transverse process fusion because it repairs the defect at one vertebral level rather than involving a second nonaffected vertebrae [134, 136]. In properly selected patients, 80–90% obtain a solid fusion with 80% good–excellent results [134, 136]. The Gill procedure or laminectomy is never indicated without an associated fusion in children [119]. Removal of the posterior elements may in fact be harmful, leading to increased instability and spondylolisthesis in the postoperative period.

References

1. Wagoner G, Pendergrass E P. The anterior and posterior "notch" shadows seen in lateral roentgenograms of the vertebrae of infants: an anatomic explanation. Am J Roentgenol. 1939;42:663–670.
2. Leventhal HR. Birth injuries of the spinal cord. J Pediatr. 1960;56:447–453.
3. Babcock JL. Spinal injuries in children. Pediatr Clin North Am. 1975;22:487–500.
4. Banniza von Bazan UK, Paeslack V. Scoliotic growth in children with acquired paraplegia [proceedings]. Paraplegia. 1977;15:65–73.
5. Glasauer FE, Cares HL. Traumatic paraplegia in infancy. JAMA. 1972;219:38–41.
6. Kewalramani LS, Tori JA. Spinal cord trauma in children. Neurologic patterns, radiologic features, and pathomechanics of injury. Spine. 1980;5:11–18.
7. Melzak J. Paraplegia among children. Lancet. 1969;2:45–48.
8. Scher AT. Trauma of the spinal cord in children. S Afr Med J. 1976;50:2023–2025.
9. Yngve DA, Harris WP, Herndon WA, et al. Spinal cord injury without osseous spine fracture. J Pediatr Orthop. 1988;8:153–159.
10. Choi JU, Hoffman HJ, Hendrick EB, et al. Traumatic infarction of the spinal cord in children. J Neurosurg. 1986;65:608–610.
11. Mayfield JK, Erkkila JC, Winter RB. Spine deformity subsequent to acquired childhood spinal cord injury. J Bone Joint Surg Am. 1981;63:1401–1411.
12. Lancourt JE, Dickson JH, Carter RE. Paralytic spinal deformity following traumatic spinal-cord injury in children and adolescents. J Bone Joint Surg Am. 1981;63:47–53.

13. McPhee IB. Spinal fractures and dislocations in children and adolescents. Spine. 1981;6:533–537.

14. Yasuoka S, Peterson HA, MacCarty CS. Incidence of spinal column deformity after multilevel laminectomy in children and adults. J Neurosurg. 1982;57:441–445.

15. Aufdermaur M. Spinal injuries in juveniles. Necropsy findings in twelve cases. J Bone Joint Surg Br. 1974;56B:513–519.

16. Hachen HJ. Spinal cord injury in children and adolescents: diagnostic pitfalls and therapeutic considerations in the acute stage [proceedings]. Paraplegia. 1977;15:55–64.

17. Hadley MN, Zabramski JM, Browner CM, et al. Pediatric spinal trauma. Review of 122 cases of spinal cord and vertebral column injuries. J Neurosurg. 1988;68:18–24.

18. Reddy SP, Junewick JJ, Backstrom JW. Distribution of spinal fractures in children: does age, mechanism of injury, or gender play a significant role? Pediatr Radiol. 2003;33:776–781.

19. Koch BM, Eng GM. Neonatal spinal cord injury. Arch Phys Med Rehabil. 1979;60:378–381.

20. Levin TL, Berdon WE, Cassell I, et al. Thoracolumbar fracture with listhesis—an uncommon manifestation of child abuse. Pediatr Radiol. 2003;33:305–310.

21. Swischuk LE. Spine and spinal cord trauma in the battered child syndrome. Radiology. 1969;92:733–738.

22. Abel MS. Transverse posterior element fractures associated with torsion. Skeletal Radiol. 1989;17:556–560.

23. Begg AC. Nuclear herniations of the intervertebral disc; their radiological manifestations and significance. J Bone Joint Surg Br. 1954;36-B:180–193.

24. Cirak B, Ziegfeld S, Knight VM, et al. Spinal injuries in children. J Pediatr Surg. 2004;39:607–612.

25. Hegenbarth R, Ebel KD. Roentgen findings in fractures of the vertebral column in childhood examination of 35 patients and its results. Pediatr Radiol. 1976;5:34–39.

26. Horal J, Nachemson A, Scheller S. Clinical and radiological long term follow-up of vertebral fractures in children. Acta Orthop Scand. 1972;43:491–503.

27. Herkowitz HN, Samberg LC. Vertebral column injuries associated with tobogganing. J Trauma. 1978;18:806–810.

28. Odom JA, Brown CW, Messner DG. Tubing injuries. J Bone Joint Surg. 1976;58A:733.

29. Shrosbree RD. Spinal cord injuries as a result of motorcycle accidents. Paraplegia. 1978;16:102–112.

30. Anderson JM, Schutt AH. Spinal injury in children: a review of 156 cases seen from 1950 through 1978. Mayo Clin Proc. 1980;55:499–504.

31. Hubbard DD. Injuries of the spine in children and adolescents. Clin Orthop. 1974:56–65.

32. Santschi M, Echave V, Laflamme S, et al. Seat-belt injuries in children involved in motor vehicle crashes. Can J Surg. 2005;48:373–376.

33. Sclafani SJ, Florence LO, Phillips TF, et al. Lumbar arterial injury: radiologic diagnosis and management. Radiology. 1987;165:709–714.

34. Sturm JT, Perry JF Jr. Injuries associated with fractures of the transverse processes of the thoracic and lumbar vertebrae. J Trauma. 1984;24:597–599.

35. Denis F. The three column spine and its significance in the classification of acute thoracolumbar spinal injuries. Spine. 1983;8:817–831.

36. Denis F. Spinal instability as defined by the three-column spine concept in acute spinal trauma. Clin Orthop. 1984:65–76.

37. Ruckstuhl J, Morscher E, Jani L. [Treatment and prognosis in vertebral fractures in children and adolescents]. Chirurg. 1976;47:458–467.

38. Roaf R. A study of the mechanics of spinal injuries. J Bone Joint Surg. 1960;42B:810–823.

39. Hubbard DD. Fractures of the dorsal and lumbar spine. Orthop Clin North Am. 1976;7:605–614.

40. Parisini P, Di Silvestre M, Greggi T. Treatment of spinal fractures in children and adolescents: long-term results in 44 patients. Spine. 2002;27:1989–1994.

41. Thomas KC, Lalonde F, O'Neil J, et al. Multiple-level thoracolumbar burst fractures in teenaged patients. J Pediatr Orthop. 2003;23:119–123.

42. Bulos S. Herniated intervertebral lumbar disc in the teenager. J Bone Joint Surg Br. 1973;55:273–278.

43. MacCartee CC Jr, Griffin PP, Byrd EB. Ruptured calcified thoracic disc in a child. Report of a case. J Bone Joint Surg Am. 1972;54:1272–1274.

44. Peck FC Jr. A calcified thoracic intervertebral disk with herniation and spinal cord compression in a child; case report. J Neurosurg. 1957;14:105–109.

45. Handel SF, Twiford TW Jr, Reigel DH, et al. Posterior lumbar apophyseal fractures. Radiology. 1979;130:629–633.

46. Keller RH. Traumatic displacement of the cartilagenous vertebral rim: a sign of intervertebral disc prolapse. Radiology. 1974;110:21–24.

47. Lippitt AB. Fracture of a vertebral body end plate and disk protrusion causing subarachnoid block in an adolescent. Clin Orthop. 1976:112–115.

48. Lowrey JJ. Dislocated lumbar vertebral epiphysis in adolescent children. Report of three cases. J Neurosurg. 1973;38:232–234.

49. Techakapuch S. Rupture of the lumbar cartilage plate into the spinal canal in an adolescent. A case report. J Bone Joint Surg Am. 1981;63:481–482.

50. Callahan DJ, Pack LL, Bream RC, et al. Intervertebral disc impingement syndrome in a child. Report of a case and suggested pathology. Spine. 1986;11:402–404.

51. Dietemann JL, Runge M, Badoz A, et al. Radiology of posterior lumbar apophyseal ring fractures: report of 13 cases. Neuroradiology. 1988;30:337–344.

52. Sovio OM, Bell HM, Beauchamp RD, et al. Fracture of the lumbar vertebral apophysis. J Pediatr Orthop. 1985;5:550–552.

53. Smith WS, Kaufer H. Patterns and mechanisms of lumbar injuries associated with lap seat belts. J Bone Joint Surg Am. 1969;51:239–254.

54. Blasier RD, LaMont RL. Chance fracture in a child: a case report with nonoperative treatment. J Pediatr Orthop. 1985;5:92–93.

55. Kolowich P, Phillips, W. Seat belt lumbar fractures in children. Orthop Trans. 1986;10:566.

56. Taylor GA, Eggli KD. Lap-belt injuries of the lumbar spine in children: a pitfall in CT diagnosis. AJR Am J Roentgenol. 1988;150:1355–1358.

57. Gumley G, Taylor TK, Ryan MD. Distraction fractures of the lumbar spine. J Bone Joint Surg Br. 1982;64:520–525.

58. Betz RR, Mulcahey MJ, D'Andrea LP, et al. Acute evaluation and management of pediatric spinal cord injury. J Spinal Cord Med. 2004;27 Suppl 1:S11–15.

59. Agran PF, Dunkle DE, Winn DG. Injuries to a sample of seatbelted children evaluated and treated in a hospital emergency room. J Trauma. 1987;27:58–64.

60. Sledge JB, Allred D, Hyman J. Use of magnetic resonance imaging in evaluating injuries to the pediatric thoracolumbar spine. J Pediatr Orthop. 2001;21:288–293.

61. Ferrandez L, Usabiaga J, Curto JM, et al. Atypical multivertebral fracture due to hyperextension in an adolescent girl. A case report. Spine. 1989;14:645–646.

62. Carreon LY, Glassman SD, Campbell MJ. Pediatric spine fractures: a review of 137 hospital admissions. J Spinal Disord Tech. 2004;17:477–482.

63. Burke DC. Spinal cord trauma in children. Paraplegia. 1971;9:1–14.

64. Burke DC. Traumatic spinal paralysis in children. Paraplegia. 1974;11:268–276.

65. Glasauer FE, Cares HL. Biomechanical features of traumatic paraplegia in infancy. J Trauma. 1973;13:166–170.

66. Betz RR, Gelman AJ, DeFilipp GJ, et al. Magnetic resonance imaging (MRI) in the evaluation of spinal cord injured children and adolescents. Paraplegia. 1987;25:92–99.

67. Akbarnia BA. Pediatric spine fractures. Orthop Clin North Am. 1999;30:521–536.

68. Boechat MI. Spinal deformities and pseudofractures. AJR Am J Roentgenol. 1987;148:97–98.

69. Gellad FE, Levine AM, Joslyn JN, et al. Pure thoracolumbar facet dislocation: clinical features and CT appearance. Radiology. 1986;161:505–508.

70. Tarr RW, Drolshagen LF, Kerner TC, et al. MR imaging of recent spinal trauma. J Comput Assist Tomogr. 1987;11:412–417.

71. McArdle CB, Crofford MJ, Mirfakhraee M, et al. Surface coil MR of spinal trauma: preliminary experience. AJNR Am J Neuroradiol. 1986;7:885–893.

72. Moller A, Hasserius R, Besjakov J, et al. Vertebral fractures in late adolescence: a 27 to 47-year follow-up. Eur Spine J. 2006;15:1247–1254.

73. Jackson RW. Surgical stabilisation of the spine. Paraplegia. 1975;13:71–74.

74. Westerborn A, Olsson, O. Mechanics, treatment and prognosis of fractures of the dorso-lumbar spine. Acta Chirurgica Scandinavica. 1953;102:59–83.

75. Lalonde F, Letts M, Yang JP, et al. An analysis of burst fractures of the spine in adolescents. Am J Orthop. 2001;30:115–120.

76. Bryant CE, Sullivan JA. Management of thoracic and lumbar spine fractures with Harrington distraction rods supplemented with segmental wiring. Spine. 1983;8:532–537.

77. Flesch JR, Leider LL, Erickson DL, et al. Harrington instrumentation and spine fusion for unstable fractures and fracture-dislocations of the thoracic and lumbar spine. J Bone Joint Surg Am. 1977;59:143–153.

78. Bradford DS, McBride GG. Surgical management of thoracolumbar spine fractures with incomplete neurologic deficits. Clin Orthop. 1987:201–216.

79. Campbell J, Bonnett C. Spinal cord injury in children. Clin Orthop. 1975:114–123.

80. Audic B, Maury M. Secondary vertebral deformities in childhood and adolescence. Paraplegia. 1969;7:11–16.

81. Bedbrook GM. Correction of scoliosis due to paraplegia sustained in paediatric age-group [proceedings]. Paraplegia. 1977;15:90–96.

82. Kilfoyle RM, Foley JJ, Norton PL. Spine and pelvic deformity in childhood and adolescent paraplegia: a study of 104 cases. J Bone Joint Surg Am. 1965;47:659–682.

83. McSweeney T. Spinal deformity after spinal cord injury. Paraplegia. 1969;6:212–221.

84. Lyons BM, Brown DJ, Calvert JM, et al. The diagnosis and management of post traumatic syringomyelia. Paraplegia. 1987;25:340–350.

85. Williams B, Terry AF, Jones F, et al. Syringomyelia as a sequel to traumatic paraplegia. Paraplegia. 1981;19:67–80.

86. Cullen JC. Spinal lesions in battered babies. J Bone Joint Surg Br. 1975;57:364–366.

87. Dickson RA, Leatherman KD. Spinal injuries in child abuse: case report. J Trauma. 1978;18:811–812.

88. Kleinman PK, Zito JL. Avulsion of the spinous processes caused by infant abuse. Radiology. 1984;151:389–391.

89. Kogutt MS, Swischuk LE, Fagan CJ. Patterns of injury and significance of uncommon fractures in the battered child syndrome. Am J Roentgenol Radium Ther Nucl Med. 1974;121: 143–149.

90. Renard M, Tridon P, Kuhnast M, et al. Three unusual cases of spinal cord injury in childhood. Paraplegia. 1978;16:130–134.

91. Carrion WV, Dormans JP, Drummond DS, et al. Circumferential growth plate fracture of the thoracolumbar spine from child abuse. J Pediatr Orthop. 1996;16:210–214.

92. Nesbit ME, Kieffer S, D'Angio GJ. Reconstitution of vertebral height in histiocytosis X: a long-term follow-up. J Bone Joint Surg Am. 1969;51:1360–1368.

93. Amstutz HC, Carey EJ. Skeletal manifestations and treatment of Gaucher's disease. Review of twenty cases. J Bone Joint Surg Am. 1966;48:670–701.

94. Ribeiro RC, Pui CH, Schell MJ. Vertebral compression fracture as a presenting feature of acute lymphoblastic leukemia in children. Cancer. 1988;61:589–592.

95. Makitie O, Doria AS, Henriques F, et al. Radiographic vertebral morphology: a diagnostic tool in pediatric osteoporosis. J Pediatr. 2005;146:395–401.

96. Ross J, Gamble J, Schultz A, et al. Back pain and spinal deformity in cystic fibrosis. Am J Dis Child. 1987;141:1313–1316.

97. Varonos S, Ansell BM, Reeve J. Vertebral collapse in juvenile chronic arthritis: its relationship with glucocorticoid therapy. Calcif Tissue Int. 1987;41:75–78.

98. Jones ET, Hensinger RN. Spinal deformity in idiopathic juvenile osteoporosis. Spine. 1981;6:1–4.

99. Sørensen HK. Scheuermann's Juvenile Kyphosis. Clinical Appearances, Radiography, Aetiology, and Prognosis. Copenhagen: Munksgaard, 1964.

100. Tribus CB. Scheuermann's kyphosis in adolescents and adults: diagnosis and management. J Am Acad Orthop Surg. 1998;6:36–43.

101. Bradford DS, Moe JH, Montalvo FJ, et al. Scheuermann's kyphosis and roundback deformity. Results of Milwaukee brace treatment. J Bone Joint Surg Am. 1974;56:740–758.

102. Blumenthal SL, Roach J, Herring JA. Lumbar Scheuermann's. A clinical series and classification. Spine. 1987;12:929–932.

103. Greene TL, Hensinger RN, Hunter LY. Back pain and vertebral changes simulating Scheuermann's disease. J Pediatr Orthop. 1985;5:1–7.

104. Scheuermann HW. The classic, kyphosis dorsalis juvenilis. Z Orthop Chir. 1921;41:305–317.

105. McCall IW, Park WM, O'Brien JP, et al. Acute traumatic intraosseous disc herniation. Spine. 1985;10:134–137.

106. Hafner RH. Localised osteochondritis (Scheuermann's disease). J Bone Joint Surg Br. 1952;34-B:38–40.

107. Micheli LJ. Low back pain in the adolescent: differential diagnosis. Am J Sports Med. 1979;7:362–364.

108. Jayson MI, Herbert CM, Barks JS. Intervertebral discs: nuclear morphology and bursting pressures. Ann Rheum Dis. 1973;32:308–315.

109. Resnick D, Niwayama G. Intravertebral disk herniations: cartilaginous (Schmorl's) nodes. Radiology. 1978;126:57–65.

110. Alexander CJ. Scheuermann's disease; a traumatic spondylodystrophy. Skeletal Radiol. 1977;1:209–221.

111. Ghelman B, Freiberger RH. The limbus vertebra: an anterior disc herniation demonstrated by discography. AJR Am J Roentgenol. 1976;127:854–855.

112. Rowe GG, Roche MB. The etiology of separate neural arch. J Bone Joint Surg Am. 1953;35-A:102–110.

113. Wertzberger KL, Peterson HA. Acquired spondylolysis and spondylolisthesis in the young child. Spine. 1980;5:437–442.

114. Wiltse LL, Newman PH, Macnab I. Classification of spondylolysis and spondylolisthesis. Clin Orthop. 1976:23–29.

115. Baker DR, McHollick W. Spondyloschisis and spondylolisthesis in children. J Bone Joint Surg. 1956;38A:933–934.

116. Hitchcock HH. Spondylolisthesis. Observations on its development, progression, and genesis. J Bone Joint Surg. 1940;22:1–16.

117. Hensinger R, Lang, JR, MacEwen, GD. Surgical management of spondylolisthesis in children and adolescents. Spine.
1976;1:207–216.

118. Sherman FC, Wilkinson RH, Hall JE. Reactive sclerosis of a pedicle and spondylolysis in the lumbar spine. J Bone Joint Surg Am.
1977;59:49–54.

119. Sherman FC, Rosenthal RK, Hall JE. Spine fusion for spondylolysis and spondylolisthesis in children. Spine. 1979;4:59–66.

120. Turner RH, Bianco AJ Jr. Spondylolysis and spondylolisthesis in children and teen-agers. J Bone Joint Surg Am.
1971;53:1298–1306.

121. Letts M, Smallman T, Afanasiev R, et al. Fracture of the pars
interarticularis in adolescent athletes: a clinical–biomechanical
analysis. J Pediatr Orthop. 1986;6:40–46.

122. Jackson DW, Wiltse LL, Cirincoine RJ. Spondylolysis in the
female gymnast. Clin Orthop. 1976:68–73.

123. Ogilvie JW, Sherman J. Spondylolysis in Scheuermann's disease.
Spine. 1987;12:251–253.

124. Libson E, Bloom RA, Shapiro Y. Scoliosis in young men with
spondylolysis or spondylolisthesis. A comparative study in symptomatic and asymptomatic subjects. Spine. 1984;9:445–447.

125. Wynne-Davies R, Scott JH. Inheritance and spondylolisthesis:
a radiographic family survey. J Bone Joint Surg Br. 1979;61-
B:301–305.

126. Fredrickson BE, Baker D, McHolick WJ, et al. The natural history of spondylolysis and spondylolisthesis. J Bone Joint Surg
Am. 1984;66:699–707.

127. Hensinger RN. Spondylolysis and spondylolisthesis in children.
Instr Course Lect. 1983;32:132–151.

128. Libson E, Bloom RA, Dinari G, et al. Oblique lumbar
spine radiographs: importance in young patients. Radiology.
1984;151:89–90.

129. Rothman SL. Computed tomography of the spine in
older children and teenagers. Clin Sports Med. 1986;5:
247–270.

130. Papanicolaou N, Wilkinson RH, Emans JB, et al. Bone scintigra-
phy and radiography in young athletes with low back pain. AJR
Am J Roentgenol. 1985;145:1039–1044.

131. van den Oever M, Merrick MV, Scott JH. Bone scintigra-
phy in symptomatic spondylolysis. J Bone Joint Surg Br.
1987;69:453–456.

132. Nachemson A. Repair of the spondylolisthetic defect and intertransverse fusion for young patients. Clin Orthop. 1976:101–105.

133. Buck JE. Direct repair of the defect in spondylolisthesis. Preliminary report. J Bone Joint Surg Br. 1970;52:
432–437.

134. Bradford DS, Iza J. Repair of the defect in spondylolysis or minimal degrees of spondylolisthesis by segmental wire fixation and
bone grafting. Spine. 1985;10:673–679.

135. Nicol RO, Scott JH. Lytic spondylolysis. Repair by wiring. Spine.
1986;11:1027–1030.

136. Pedersen AK, Hagen R. Spondylolysis and spondylolisthesis.
Treatment by internal fixation and bone-grafting of the defect.
J Bone Joint Surg Am. 1988;70:15–24.

Index